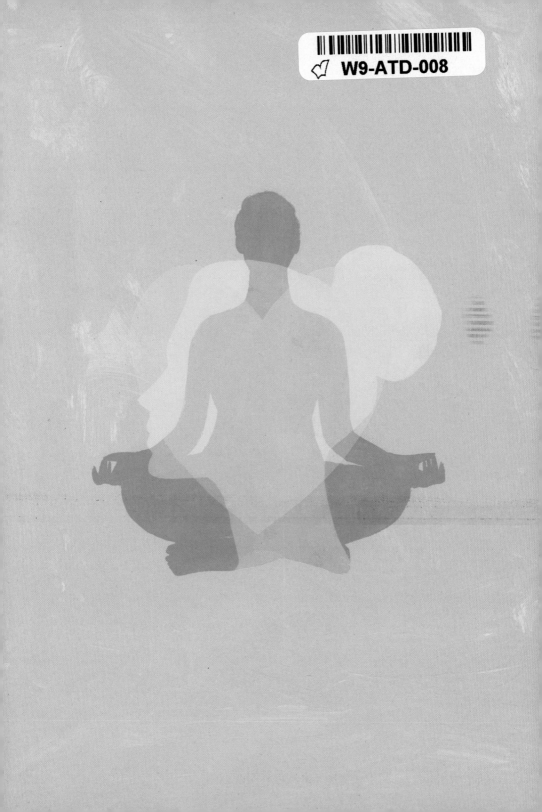

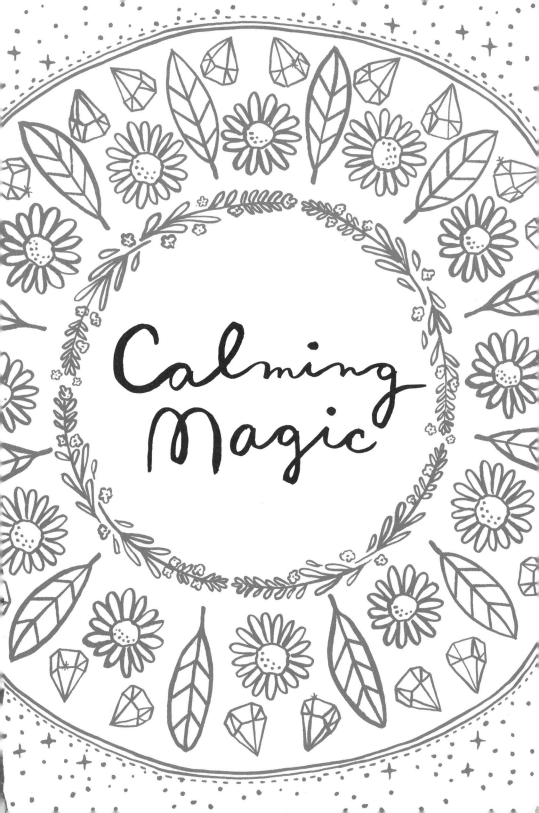

Calming Magic

Running Press
Hachette Book Group
1290 Avenue of the Americas, New York, NY 10104
www.runningpress.com
@Running_Press

Printed in China

First Edition: September 2020

Published by Running Press, an imprint of Perseus Books, LLC, a subsidiary
of Hachette Book Group, Inc. The Running Press name and logo is a trademark
of the Hachette Book Group.

The Hachette Speakers Bureau provides a wide range of authors for
speaking events. To find out more, go to www.hachettespeakersbureau.com
or call (866) 376-6591.

The publisher is not responsible for websites (or their content) that
are not owned by the publisher.

Print book cover and interior design by Susan Van Horn.

Library of Congress Control Number: 2020935027

ISBNs: 978-0-7624-7046-4 (hardcover), 978-0-7624-7047-1 (ebook)

1010

10 9 8 7 6 5 4 3 2 1

Calming Magic

ENCHANTED RITUALS FOR PEACE, CLARITY, AND CREATIVITY

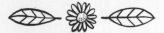

NIKKI VAN DE CAR

illustrations by
PENELOPE DULLAGHAN

RUNNING PRESS
PHILADELPHIA

CONTENTS

Creativity

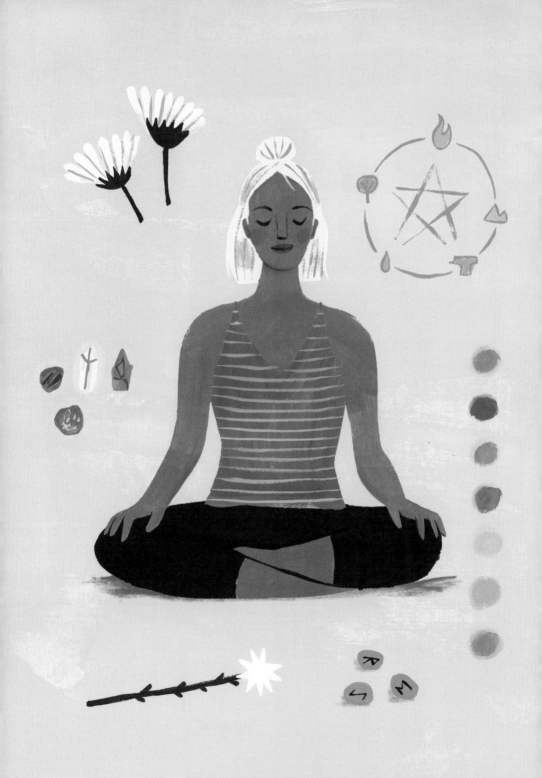

INTRODUCTION

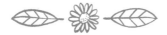

THESE ARE CHALLENGING TIMES. Between politics, health crises, family dramas, and the everyday irritants at work, we can often feel besieged by life. It may seem like there is a vast conspiracy bent on keeping our blood pressure up, our nights sleepless, and our hearts heavy. And the reality is that those stressors are real and, for the most part, aren't going anywhere. While we take steps to work more productively, take breaks from news cycles, live a healthy lifestyle, and set positive boundaries with those we love, none of that will allow us to live a completely stress-free life. From time to time, life is just *hard*, and it feels that way.

But life isn't *just* hard. Life at the same time is joyful, passionate, creative, peaceful, and—yes—magical. That magic is *always* available to you, even in your most difficult moments. We can find magic in a breeze carrying the scent of the ocean, in laughter, in a delicious meal. We can find magic by connecting to the natural world, our creativity, and the power of the feminine. The rituals, spells, and practices in this book will offer you the means to reconnect to the magic of living.

There are so many different paths to a place of magic. Cultures around the world have created their own maps and their own methods for harnessing the energies of the earth—an enduring source of peace, calm, and wonder. This book will by no means touch on all of them, but instead provide a guide to the power of feng shui, crystal healing, runic magic, chakras,

1

tarot, moon magic, yoga, herb magic, and more. It will give you anything and everything you need to keep your mind calm and heart open in a mad world. And specific sections on each of these powerful magics dot the book, growing your knowledge as you practice the rituals and spells.

But it won't leave you there, because there is more to life than peace. We cannot exist detached from all that is around us—we also have to engage with our experiences with clarity and creativity in order to truly *live*. Once you have the tools you need to create a calm space, you can practice looking more closely—both at the world around you and within yourself—for that is often where the answers to our most profound questions lie. The same pathways you will be using to find calm will open you up to insight, as you employ celestite to help you view a problem through eyes unclouded by the fog of your emotions or turn to tarot to aid you in uncovering what it is that you truly want in life. Throughout this book, you'll be prompted to take a moment to journal and write down any insights you've received. Sometimes the simple act of putting pen to paper brings release, clarity, and a sense of purpose.

For once you know what it is you want, you can go about getting it. We are responsible for generating the life we want to live, but so often the power of that creativity gets lost in the weight of our burdens. All those things that have caused us to lose our sense of calm in the first place—the everyday stressors, the fears for the future of our planet, the emotional roller coaster that is a life shared with other people—are things that can sever us from our own creativity and inherent power. But the same rituals, spells, and mystical skills that will bring you peace and insight will assist you in regaining your power to live every day with joy, purpose . . . and even magic.

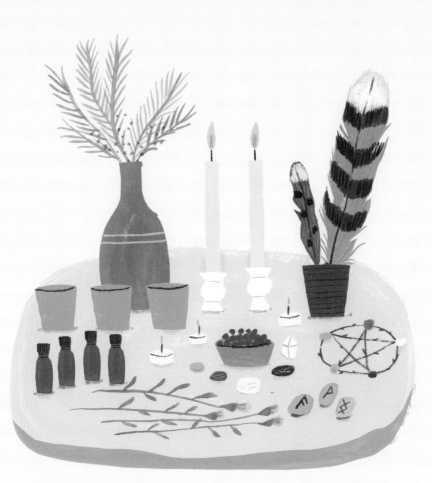

About Altars

Although altars are one of those things that may feel a little "out there" or even just a little too religious, an altar is just a simple, practical way of connecting with your own spirituality on a daily basis by making it a **part** of your life. While it's true that altars often incorporate religious texts, symbols, and deities, they don't have to. They can function kind of like an ongoing spell, without beginning or end. They are a place to focus your thoughts and energies in either very specific or very general ways, depending on what's going on in your life at that moment.

3

An altar isn't necessarily for prayer or worship, though it certainly can be. At heart, it's a space dedicated to your connection to *something more*—that thing people call Source or God or the Universe or Energy. You can use whatever word resonates for you, or no word at all, but your altar is the place where you interact with it and honor it. We are physical beings, and as such we connect on a physical level—even with what is metaphysical.

There are no rules for creating this physical space. It is entirely under your control and something that you can evolve over time. That said, setting up an altar can feel a little intimidating at first, so here are some general guidelines:

LOCATION. Depending on your lifestyle, you can keep your altar out in the open in a living room or entryway, but if you've got a lot people coming in and out and you want to keep this part of yourself a little more private, you can create an altar in your bedroom. You can use a part of the top of your dresser or bedside table or find a small bench to place in a corner of the room. You don't need a lot of space; a square foot or more is usually sufficient.

CENTRAL SYMBOL. Often, an altar has a focus, though again, it doesn't have to. There are no "have-tos" here! But you might want to consider placing a large, powerful crystal or a photograph or some other image at the center of your altar. This can be of someone you love, an ancestor or goddess, or a place that has meaning for you. You could use a bowl or chalice if you want to focus on inviting positive energies into your life or an incense burner if you want to disperse negative energies. Whatever feels right *is* right, and you can rearrange or reinvent your altar at any time.

ELEMENTS. You may also want to consider incorporating four or five powerful elements. As discussed on page 7, feng shui embraces fire, earth, water, and metal, but other traditions often include air in place of metal.

- **Fire:** You could use a candle, volcanic stones, or some incense.

- **Water:** You could use a seashell, a mirror, or a jar of rainwater or river water.

- **Earth:** You could use horn or bone, sedimentary rock or pottery.

- **Air:** You could use a feather, an essential oil diffuser, or some eggshells.

- **Metal:** You could use a ring or pendant you feel an emotional connection to or a chain or bell.

PERSONAL ITEMS. Pieces of friendship bracelets, lost keys, buttons, crystals, dried herbs—be like a magpie! The most powerful parts of your altar are likely items that would be meaningless to anyone else, but that speak to you on a soul level.

USING YOUR ALTAR

An altar is meaningless unless you have a relationship with it. If you create it and then let it sit there gathering dust, all you have is a pretty collection of knick-knacks. It doesn't take much to keep an altar alive: feeding and watering it can be as simple as glancing at it once or twice a day. Rearranging it can recharge it, and meditating over it can bring you a deeper form of mindfulness.

But to get the most impact out of your altar, make it a part of your daily life. There are specific practices for deeper altar work in this book, but it is simple enough to create an everyday ritual that will enhance the synergetic power you have with your altar. If you've included incense or a candle in your sacred space, take the time every day to light it and sit with it. If you've included an image of an inspiration or a loved one, take a moment to speak with them, even if it's only a nod of recognition. You can pull a tarot card for the day and leave it faceup on your altar, keeping its energy present there throughout the day.

You may also consider leaving offerings at your altar on occasion. This needn't be done on a daily basis, but rather in times of hardship or when you're feeling of service to others or to the world. Some fruit, a small found item, a glass of wine—again, whatever feels right. You should clear away the offering when it feels right, too—and you should feel free to eat the fruit or drink the wine! Your altar is a space you share with *something more*.

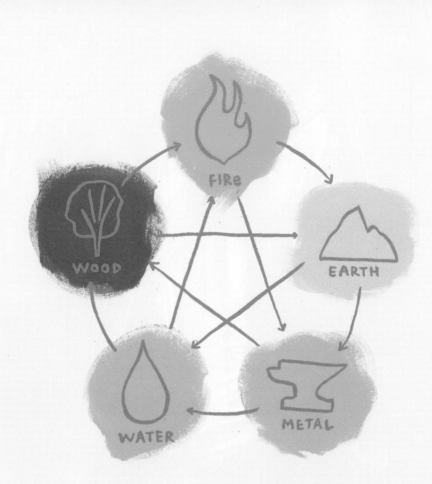

About Feng Shui

Feng shui is the simple practice of bringing your surroundings into harmony with nature. In this case, nature is defined as your own, internal nature and as the natural world. Feng shui is a form of *geomancy*, or divination through interpreting the natural world. That means that astrology is another form of geomancy, as are dowsing, rune-casting, and the I Ching. But feng shui's geomancy is less about reading the *signs* of nature and more about using the *elements* of nature to impact our lives. The practice began as ancient Chinese geomancers studied the patterns of the elements and learned how they could be harnessed, instead of just interpreted.

There are three core principles at work within feng shui: the elements, qi—which translates to "energy or life-force" and is essentially the same thing as prana, as discussed on page 48—and the bagua, which is a map of your space, featuring principles like abundance, career, family, and so forth—all the things we navigate throughout our lives.

Qi in feng shui refers not just to your own energy, but also to the inherent energy of the things that surround you. We imbue objects with energy. Consider a stuffed animal that you still hang on to. It's faded and probably falling apart, but you would never throw it away. Or look at the blanket you've had since college. It's a little stained, maybe it even has some holes in it, but it's still the softest and warmest blanket you own—or it feels like it anyway. This is positive, free-flowing qi. On the other hand, there are objects that block the flow of qi. Sometimes we're given gifts we feel we ought to like, but don't. So a painting or a lamp your aunt bought you is on display, but it makes you feel a little uneasy. Or perhaps you bought yourself a slow cooker because you meant to use it, but it just sits there on the counter gathering dust—that's blocked qi, too. If you can open up these blocks, either reevaluating your feelings and intentions around the items in your home or simply redecorating, you can move that qi around so that it flows in a peaceful, natural rhythm.

The baguas are a way to help you figure out how to keep those flows moving and draw more qi into a certain aspect of your life when you need to.

The baguas are divided into the four cardinal directions—south, west, north, and east—as well as the intermediate southwest, northwest, northeast, and southeast. Each of these directions represents an area in your home, and an aspect of your life. The center of the bagua—and the center of your home—represents a healthy state, where all of your elements, and all of the different demands you place on yourself, are in balance.

Now, most of our houses are not octagonal, so this diagram is a very rough guide. You can use the bagua in whatever way feels the most natural to you. If there is a room in a northern part of your house that would make a good home office, terrific! If you can put your kitchen in the eastern side, that's great, too.

8

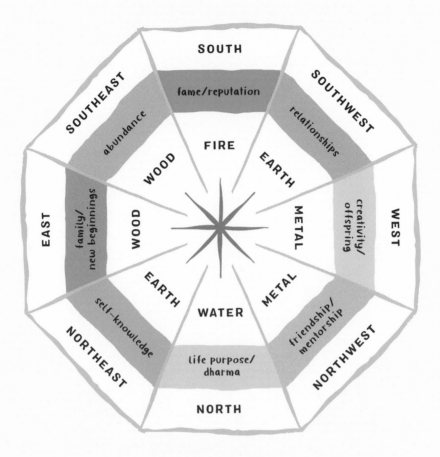

And if some of these parts of life feel less important to you than others—so if fame is less important than health and creativity, for example—then feel free to minimize that. You also don't have to align your bagua with the cardinal directions. This is the traditional method, but it has since been updated to work without taking the directions into account, but instead adapting to a natural flow that works with the layout of your house. Whatever feels right for you is right for you. This is about your qi, your space, and should reflect you.

The term *feng shui* translates to "wind-water," highlighting two of the five elements (fire, earth, wood, water, and metal) that the art holds in balance. Each element resonates with a particular section of the bagua, and in feng shui, each element is called forth by a specific shape or color, as well as its literal self—so water can be represented by a fountain, but also by a mirror or a dark-colored painting.

FIRE

We have to be a little cautious with fire. Fire is joyful, energetic, and transformative, but it can also be destructive. There can be too much of a good thing, but as long as you pay attention to the impact fire has on you, its brightness and heat can bring you more energy, allowing your life to contain more passion and you to perhaps even experience powerful changes for the better. Candles and lamps are the most obvious way to incorporate more fire into your home, but you can also highlight the color red, as well as anything triangular or pointed. Fire sets alight your fame and reputation bagua sector, as well as bringing more heat to the marriage and relationships sector.

EARTH

The element of earth represents stability and feeling grounded. It has the same energy as your root chakra (see page 49). It is the base for all the other elements and for your entire life, and every home should have plenty of earth represented in it.

Contrary, perhaps, to our modern expectations, earth's shape in feng shui is square and flat, though this might make a little more sense when we remember that the principles of feng shui date back for centuries to a time before we knew the earth is round. Pottery and other ceramics are a great way to ground your space in earth, and in lieu of that, you can incorporate yellow into your decor, perhaps in a square floor pillow or an area rug—something low to the ground, stable and warm. Earth nourishes two of the most important bagua centers in your home: your relationships with others and your relationship with yourself.

WOOD

• The wood element helps promote growth and creativity. If you're looking to expand your intuition, be more imaginative, or grow as a person, incorporating some wood into your home will move that process along. That can be as simple as buying a houseplant or making something out of driftwood. Wood is represented by the color green, as well as anything tall and vertical. Thin, rectangular shapes will call forth the element of wood. On the bagua map, wood can be found in new beginnings/family and abundance: parts of our lives that always need nurturing and growth.

WATER

Water represents sanctuary, healing, and spirituality—but also a lack of structure and a sense of the unknown. Consider how we depend on water literally for life, but also have no way of predicting it. It flows where it will, sometimes smoothly and calmly and sometimes violently. Water is not the destructive force that fire is, but it does ask you to be comfortable with a little uncertainty. Think of water less as a clear glass of liquid and more like the reflection you see when you peer into a lake or a river: it's a little distorted, a little mysterious.

Mirrors and other reflective surfaces represent water, as do dark colors and blues. Unlike the other elements, water is not attached to a specific shape, but instead is brought to mind by anything sinuous and flowing. Long curtains blowing in the breeze or a blanket thrown across an armchair can represent water. Water is in the life purpose/dharma section of the bagua, which, again, may be counterintuitive. Perhaps it feels like wood or fire could fuel life purpose better than gentle water ever could. But consider how we must grow calm and look deep within in order to truly know our life purpose—for dharma is not just something we do, it's something we are.

METAL

If you're feeling indecisive and unstructured, it's probably a good idea to introduce more metal into your surroundings. Metal is the hardest of all the elements, and it will help you make reasoned, considered choices, stick to a schedule, and make a clear plan.

The shape of the metal element is a circle, and its color is a shiny, nonreflective gray, so a silver-plated vase or round picture frame is an excellent way to add metal to your home. You can also include gray, round throw pillows, or, if you want a more widespread essence of metal rather than a single eye-catching piece, you can paint a room gray. Metal is found in the creativity/offspring section, as well as the friendship/mentorship section of the bagua. It may seem odd at first to think about creativity relating to structured metal, but it makes sense—unstructured creativity never comes to fruition, and metal is all about making sure things happen the way you want them to. And well, having some structure in your friendships and your relationships with your children is always a good idea. These are people that depend on us, and they are aided by the kind of careful attention brought forth by metal.

BALANCING THE ELEMENTS

The elements are all in relationship with each other, and they create cycles as they interact. There are two forms of cycles: constructive and destructive. In a constructive cycle, the elements are enhancing and complementing one another, making each other stronger.

* Water nurtures wood.
* Wood feeds fire.
* Fire enhances earth.

* Earth forms metal.
* Metal intensifies water.

So if you're looking to boost a particular element, you should also use the element that complements it. If you want to bring more fire into your life, wood will make it burn more brightly. And since ashes turn to dirt, fire feeds earth. Earth over time compacts into metal, which dissolves in water.

On the other hand, from time to time you may want to lessen the impact of a particular element, and here is where the destructive cycle can come into play.

* Water dowses fire.
* Fire weakens metal.
* Metal cuts wood.

* Wood consumes earth.
* Earth stops water.

If you want to allow the passion of fire into your home, but also temper and control it, balance it with some water. If you need to feel a little more grounded and a little less mysterious, stop the flow of water with earth. Allow more creativity with the new growth that is wood, as its heights stretch away from the ground, but control that wood with the structure of metal.

ᚠᚢᚦᚨᚱᚲᚷ

ᚹᚺᚾᛁᛃᛇᛈ

ᛉᛊᛏᛒᛖᛗ

ᛚᛜᛟᛞ

About Runes

There are several different varieties of runes, from several different places around the world. They were originally a system of writing for various Germanic languages before the Latin alphabet gained dominance. The Elder Futhark specifically dates back to the second century and was thought to be used not just for communication, but also for divination, protection, and other forms of magic. The word *rune* translates to "secret," and only the wisest and bravest would attempt to interpret or use them. If you were, say, a Viking chieftain and needed some advice on whether the seas were fair for exploration, you would consult with your *erilaz* (sorcerer advisor), who would cast the runes onto a cloth and entreat them to determine the best course of action.

The truth is, there isn't much in the way of direct evidence that runes were employed for divination, though divination is the most common use for runes today. There isn't much in the way of direct evidence of what runes were used for at all—or anything about what life was like so long ago for that matter. More than anything, all that we have are the stories we tell, the stories that were passed down to us from the ones who were there. Did some things change in the telling and retelling? Probably, but it is through stories that we understand ourselves and the world around us, and these stories have informed how we approach and use runes.

Because of this murky history, you can find varying interpretations behind each of the runes. Since we don't know precisely what they meant, we have all told different stories about them. And in fact, as you work with them, you will come to tell your own stories and give them your own meanings—that flexibility is part of their magic. Runes were—and still are—carved onto stone tiles, which are typically kept in a small cloth bag. They can be used as an oracle, much in the way you would work with a tarot deck. But rune-casting is much simpler, though much more open to interpretation. You will need a cloth for casting—typically a white cloth, but it doesn't truly matter. You just need something that will create a boundary for your runes and hold them so you can read them.

FEHU (Cattle)

It's a rune of abundance, luck, and energy. It represents new beginnings and the ability to create wealth—be it monetary or simply the means to live in the way that you want to. It also urges you to safeguard this wealth, as it was not easily won.

ANSUZ (Divine breath)

Ansuz represents divine order and stability. It also aids in communication, as it asks you to listen while knowing that you too will be heard.

URUZ (Aurochs; wild ox)

This is a call to be wild, to push beyond your boundaries. It asks for determination, even stubbornness, and can be used for healing as well.

RAIDHO (Journey)

As the Vikings were adventurers and explorers, so too can you be. But doing so takes planning and careful thought, for this is not a journey to be undertaken lightly.

THURISAZ (Giant, thorns)

This rune asks you to protect yourself and can provide protection. Chaos may be at hand, but you can hunker down and stay out of the coming storm.

KENAZ (Torch)

A rune of knowledge and inspiration, Kenaz asks you to strive for learning and perfect your skills with creativity, putting yourself into your work.

GEBO (Gift)

This can mean generosity, a literal gift, but it is also a reminder that when you live among others, gifts cannot stand alone: what you receive, you should give elsewhere in return.

NAUTHIZ (Necessity)

There is work that needs to be done, and it isn't work we want to be doing. It may come in a time of hardship, where we learn the lessons we need to move toward the promise of Fehu.

WUNJO (Joy)

This kind of joy can come through desire and romantic love, but also through contentment and harmony. Wunjo can dissipate pain and suffering and is an indication that good things are coming your way.

ISA (Ice)

This rune is about stillness and concentration, but also about feeling stuck—when it appears, it indicates that everything is grinding to a halt. But you can use this forced rest to see what you might've been missing in the rush.

HAGALAZ (Hail)

This is a difficult storm. It is a crisis, even a catastrophe, and like hailstones it will hurt. But while hailstorms come on suddenly, often without warning, they do pass quickly and melt away without much lasting damage.

JERA (Harvest)

This rune represents the cycle of life, how we continue onward and forward always. There is a sense of peace in that.

EIHWAZ (Yew tree)

A rune of birth and death, symbolizing new beginnings. It can be used for protection and power during transitions.

SOWILO (Sun)

A guide to finding light in dark times. Sowilo invites strength, confidence, and a sense of wholeness. There has been a struggle, but you are finding your way through.

PERTHRO (Fate)

This rune is hard to interpret, as it represents secrets and the unknown—that which cannot be grasped, but still influences us. When it appears, it is a reminder that there are forces beyond our control, but we should do our best with what we *can* control.

TIWAZ (Creator)

When this rune appears, it is a call to sacrifice. You may find that the answer is to choose the greater good—it is the right thing to do.

ALGIZ (Elk)

This rune symbolizes our connection with the gods. When it appears, it is a call to listen to your intuition, and it can also be used as a protective talisman.

BERKANO (Birch tree)

This is a rune of creativity and fertility. It harnesses all the aspects of feminine power: insight, healing, nurturing, and rebirth.

EHWAZ (Horse)

A horse represents freedom, motion, and independence, but also cooperation, for you must learn to work together to get where you want to go.

INGUZ (Seed).

This rune of creativity and fertility is about internal work, about creating a force within yourself before sharing it with others.

MANNAZ (Humankind)

Mannaz is about the importance of community, of responsibility to others and the joys of living in harmony. It is also a rune of intelligence.

OTHALA (Household).

This is about your home and hearth, and the comfort and protection they provide. But it is also about your family, including your ancestors, and what you have inherited from them.

LAGUZ (Water)

Water contains multitudes—life, dreams, mystery, imagination, and emotion. It is our source, and we cannot live without it, though we will never entirely understand it.

DAGAZ (Dawn)

Dawn represents the balance between the light and the dark. We can, and must, hold both within us at all times, for only then can we live as we truly are.

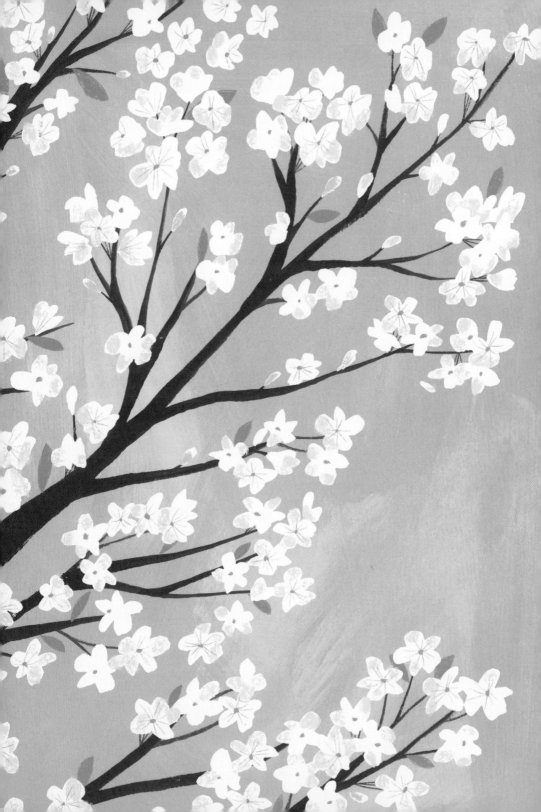

PEACE
freedom from disturbance, tranquility

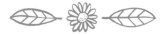

THE TRUTH IS THAT TRUE PEACE IS A RARE EXPERIENCE.

Imagine your most peaceful moment: You are lying in an open field, beneath the branches of a blossoming cherry tree. The air is warm, but there is a gentle breeze keeping you cool. You close your eyes and watch the light flicker beyond your eyelids as the sun peeks through the flowers.

It's wonderful. And yet, there's a fly landing on your ankle. You twitch it away. You suddenly remember an email you forgot to send, and you frown. There's nothing you can do about it now, but the thought is there. A truck rumbles by on the road near the field, disturbing the silence.

These things will happen. Trucks will be loud, insects will annoy, and our minds never really stop working away. The trick is to find peace anyway—the peace that exists beside those disturbances. We live in the world and the world is not perfectly tranquil, but peace does exist and can be found amid all its multifaceted experiences.

The practices in this section draw on serene magic and are intended to help you find peace within and around those distractions and stressors—even in moments that are decidedly not peaceful.

Body

Root Chakra Practice

We cannot feel calm unless we feel safe. Muladhara, the root chakra, governs that feeling of safety. It is the source of the sense of being grounded, of knowing we aren't going to fly apart. Without it, nothing else is possible. To unblock your root chakra, begin by gathering crystals that will resonate with muladhara: obsidian, hematite, agate, bloodstone, bronzite, or smoky quartz. These physical objects contain mystical properties that will aid you in your quest for calm. You will need a total of five stones.

Sit cross-legged on the earth or the floor if you can't get out of doors. Place one crystal beneath each of your hips. You don't have to sit on the crystals—that could be quite uncomfortable. Instead, place them just where your legs rise up from the earth, nestling them so that you can feel them against you, but they aren't pressing into you. Place one crystal in each of the hollows at the top of your hips. Hold your final crystal in the palm of one hand, cupping the other hand beneath it to support it. Close your hands into a fist, one that is tight, but not clenched—just firm and contained. Lower your fist to your lap.

If you'd like to chant, the sound associated with muladhara is LAM, pronounced "lum." But if chanting makes you feel exposed or uncomfortable, don't do it. You can imagine the sound in your mind, if you like, or you can imagine a song that brings you comfort. It might be something sung to you as a child like "You Are My Sunshine."

22

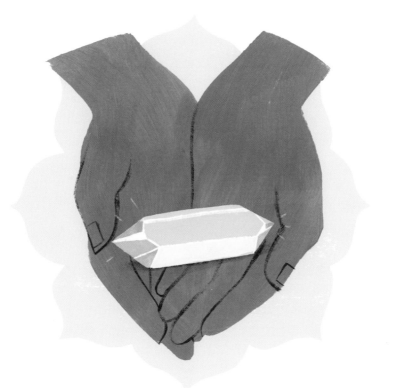

Remember the feeling of safety you had when you were young, of being carried and held. Imagine that sense of security like a roof over your head, sheltering you. Imagine the voice of a parent or someone who has always protected and cared for you. Remember them helping you back up when you fell, and recall the feeling of their hand in yours as you crossed the street.

Now, transform that sense of assurance from outside yourself into your own. You have crossed the street on your own for a while now, often ignoring crosswalks. You know what to watch out for. That caring, that protection you receive from others hasn't gone away—they still love and are there for you. But you also have the ability to protect yourself. You do it all the time, without even thinking about it.

Feel how warm the crystals have grown against your skin. Feel their heat, and know that it is your own.

Softening Lotion

This recipe is adapted from herbalist Rosemary Gladstar. It is gentle enough to use on the face—though you only need a small amount—and if kept cool, it will go for months and months without spoiling. The aloe, coconut, and almond oil will soothe and detox the skin, while the calendula, chamomile, and rose are all imbued with properties that will gently soothe the spirit, as well.

Over very low heat, combine

- ¾ cup almond oil

- ⅓ cup coconut oil

- ½ ounce beeswax

Once the oils have melted, set them aside, letting them come to room temperature. While the mixture is cooling, pull out your blender and combine:

- ⅔ cup purified water

- ⅓ cup aloe vera gel

- 2 drops calendula essential oil

- 2 drops chamomile essential oil

- 2 drops rose essential oil

Turn on your blender and mix. Then, slowly add the oils, just a bit at a time. Once the oils have been added, let the blender run on high for a few minutes, though watch it carefully. Once your ingredients begin to look like the consistency of buttercream frosting, it's time to turn it off.

Pour your lotion into jars. Store the jars you aren't currently using in the refrigerator, or give them away as gifts.

Soothing Tea

Begin by calming your insides. We carry so much stress within us, and it seeps into our bones, our blood, the molecules that form us. This tea will soothe from the inside out, relaxing your muscles and helping your adrenal system realize that it doesn't need to be in overdrive, not right now. It can take a break.

Gather a combination of dried yarrow, vervain, lemon balm, chamomile, and rue. All of these plants are common in herbal medicine and are known to promote tranquility. You only need a teaspoon in total for just one cup of tea, so create a blend according to what you have on hand, and what scents and tastes appeal to you. Put on a pot of water to boil, and turn it off once the bubbles have started. Let it come to rest, and then pour it over your tea strainer. Allow your tea to steep for five minutes.

While it's steeping, cup it in your palms, or simply lean over it if the mug is too hot. Close your eyes and inhale its fragrance.

As you breathe, your thoughts will drift to the things that disturb your calm. That's natural, we all do that. It's okay to let them. These thoughts are there, inside you, and there's no point in pretending they aren't. If you ignore them, they tend to shout to get your attention, so let them be heard. But then inhale the tea, and let your breath drift gently toward those thoughts, imagining surrounding and calming them. Let them flow out through you, magically drawing out of your body with your exhale.

Once your tea has finished steeping, take a sip. It should be cool enough. Feel your tea flow down your throat, into your belly. Sense its warmth spread through your entire body, soothing and relaxing you.

Yin Yoga

Yin yoga is a fairly recent term in the world of yoga, though the practice itself has been around for centuries. As opposed to more dynamic practices like flow or hatha yoga, here we go at a much gentler pace, moving from one pose to another slowly and smoothly and holding those poses for a much longer period of time—often three to five minutes. This method invites both strength and ease in the body, allowing the body to do the work of relaxing into a pose, rather than being forced into it through motion.

This can feel weird at first. If you're used to an asana practice, just hanging out in a single pose and not really doing anything can feel uncomfortable. You can sense those disturbances coming up with nothing to distract you from them. But again, when you distract yourself, they just start to yell louder to get your attention. Yin yoga provides an opportunity to listen to those disturbances, and then soothe them, so that you can find true calm within. As your muscles release with the forces of gravity and patience, your tension will fall away.

UTTANASANA
(Forward Fold)

From a standing position, with your feet hip-width apart, fold forward. Bend your knees generously, allowing your belly to touch the tops of your thighs. Let the weight of your upper body and head release toward the earth. Let the blood flow toward your head, and imagine all the things you want to let go of flowing out of you into the earth. You can let your fingertips fall to the earth, and sway back and forth, drawing your hands in an arc around your feet, like you're brushing your fingers through blades of grass, brushing the thoughts away. They are no longer needed.

ANAHATASANA

UTTANASANA

GOMUKHASANA

BADDHA KONASANA

JATHARA
PARIVARTANASANA

ANAHATASANA

(Heart to Earth Pose)

Start on your hands and knees, and then walk your knees back behind you, arching your hips up toward the sky. Lower your elbows to the earth, keeping your arms and legs parallel, like railroad tracks. Gently allow your head and heart to touch the earth. As you rest here, feel the bend in your upper back. Allow the thoughts to come. When you think of something that hurts your heart, focus on your heartbeat as it presses again and again into the mat. When your mind feels distracted, feel your forehead press down, and perhaps rock your head from side to side, massaging your third eye. Remind yourself that your body can feel at ease.

GOMUKHASANA

(Cow Face Pose)

Return to your hands and knees and cross one knee behind the other. Sink backward onto your sit bones, and adjust so that both hips are flat on the ground and one knee is resting on top of the other. You'll likely need to move your feet and wiggle around a bit to get comfortable and grounded. Place one palm on top of the other and rest them on your knees. Don't press down, just let the weight of your hands—which isn't very much weight at all—remind your knees to drift downward, opening the hips. If you'd like a deeper stretch, hinge forward at the hips, curving your spine over your knees. Breathe here, feeling the stretch in your back and the release in your hips.

BADDHA KONASANA

(Butterfly Pose)

Fold a blanket over several times, or grab a pillow and rest it under your hips, elevating them slightly above your knees. Bring the soles of your feet together and open your knees wide, opening your hips in the opposite direction. Don't force your knees down toward the floor—remember, gravity is doing the work here, not you. As you rest in the pose, your hips will loosen, and you won't need to hold your knees up. As you rest, rub your toes, the soles of your feet. Your feet do so much for you—they carry you everywhere you go. Give them a little love. If you like, you can lean forward, using your elbows to help your hips to release . . . or not.

JATHARA PARIVARTANASANA

(Reclined Twist)

Lie flat on your back and bring one knee up to your chest. Guide your knee to the opposite side of your mat, feeling your lower body twist. Let your knee come to the earth, and let gravity pull your opposite shoulder back to earth as well. Feel those opposing forces, sinking both sides of your body into the mat. Sense the twist in your spine, as if you are wringing yourself out like a towel. Rinse and repeat on the other side.

Restful Balm

The most important thing you can do to find a sense of peace and calm is to gift yourself with a good night's restorative sleep.

This is of course easier said than done. We are a culture of insomniacs, and we don't help ourselves. We know we ought to turn off Netflix and put away our phones. We know we ought to skip that extra glass of wine after dinner, and we know we ought to get plenty of exercise. And yes, we should definitely do all of that—but sometimes it isn't enough. Sometimes we need the promise of a little something extra, a little intention and, yes, a little magic to help us find that gentle rest.

- ¼ cup oil (olive, almond, jojoba, or another carrier oil of your choice)
- ½ cup combination of lavender, chamomile, lemon balm, and valerian, fresh or dried
- ¼ oz beeswax, grated
- 15 drops lavender essential oil
- 10 drops chamomile essential oil
- Small jar

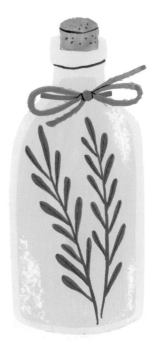

Start by creating an herbal oil. Chop or bruise your chosen herbs and place them in a small jar. Fill the jar with the carrier oil of your choice, covering the herbs by one inch and leaving one inch of space at the top. Close the jar tightly, and allow it to sit in as much sunshine as possible for a month. The heat of the sun will allow the herbs to release their juices, and infuse your blend with its powerful magic. Bring your jar indoors on moonlit nights, as the moon may stimulate more mental activity during sleep than you really want at this time, and surround it with bismuth or sapphire to promote tranquility.

When the month has passed, strain the oil through a cheesecloth and heat it over very low heat just until you can feel the warmth rising. Add the beeswax and stir clockwise until it has melted. As it is melting, clean your jar. Remove from the heat and pour the mixture back into the clean jar. Add your essential oils and stir. Cover and let it set for at least two hours before using.

When you feel you need it, rub this balm gently on your chest and the soles of your feet before you climb into bed.

Heart Chakra Practice

Before you begin, sit with your heart a moment. Are you feeling overly emotional, or are you feeling cut off, hardened by the world? When anahata, the heart chakra, is overactive, your emotions can run rampant, so that you overreact to everything and the smallest troubles will feel enormous. But a blocked heart chakra, one that stops you from actually feeling your emotions, isn't good either, because it's not like those emotions don't exist—they're always there—and they can run amok and wreak havoc with your life and your body if you don't pay attention to them. To find the balance of your emotions, begin by gathering some crystals that resonate with anahata, including rose quartz, morganite, malachite, emerald, or rhodonite. If you have a few choices, sit with each of them for a moment. Hold each and rub it between your fingers or against your cheek. The heart knows what it wants—which crystal feels the most comforting to you, the most loving? That is the one you should work with today.

Kneel on a yoga mat, pillow, or rolled-up towel. Cup your chosen crystal in your left hand and place it against your heart. Cover your left hand with your right. Bow your head and close your eyes. Cave your body in around your heart, curling your shoulders and rounding the spine. Fold over your knees. Take a breath here.

Then, roll up. Rise up on your knees and arch your back, lifting your heart up to the sky. Don't overdo it here, just allow your shoulder blades to come together like wings and your heart to open like a book. Take a breath.

Slowly, curl back down, back into your protected cave. Take another breath, and then expand up again, this time releasing your breath with a chanted YAM, pronounced "yummmmmmmmm."

Repeat three or four more times, flowing in and out, up and down. This is how your emotions should move. They come, and then they recede, and we allow them to do so. We don't fight them, as they will only fight us back. We find balance within the ebb and flow of our emotions, as we give and receive love.

Come back to a kneeling position, upright. Release your palms from your chest and allow them to fall open on your lap, with your crystal still held gently in your palm. Breathe in, and then out, feeling the ebb and flow of your breath.

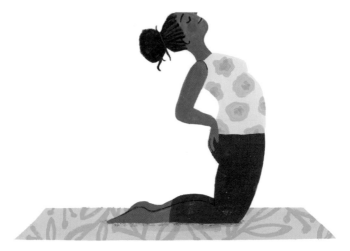

Mind

Altar Practice

Your altar is something that you should interact with every day, and it should change as you do and reflect what it is that you need. If your mind is in need of more peace, then your altar is the place to start. This is the center of your magical practice and a place of respite and rejuvenation.

Begin by doing a little cleanup. It's hard to feel at peace when things are messy and disorganized. Do some dusting, straightening, and even rearranging. It'll settle your thoughts as you begin to consider what to add or subtract. Then, take a look at each piece of your altar. Do you have a picture or object that symbolizes something you want to achieve? If so, you might want to put it away for a little while. Setting it aside for the moment doesn't mean you won't ever achieve it or even that you don't want to anymore—it's more about allowing yourself to remove the pressure of that goal. Sometimes pressure is good—we wouldn't get anywhere without it. But sometimes it isn't worth it.

Is there anything else that should be put away for a while? If your centerpiece is an incense holder or candle, maybe that isn't the right energy for you right now. Maybe an amethyst, aquamarine, or moonstone crystal would serve you better. Maybe an image of a peaceful place or a bowl of water fits your mood at this time.

Take a moment to place some items that bring you a sense of calm—perhaps some soft wool or a piece of moss. Write out a scrap of poem, like "'Hope' Is The Thing with Feathers" by Emily Dickinson:

Hope is the thing with feathers
That perches in the soul -
And sings th tune without the words -
And never stops - at all -

And sweetest - in the Gale - is heard
And sore must be the storm -
That could abash the little Bird
That kept so many warm -

I've heard it in the chillest land -
And on the strangest Sea -
Yet - never - in Extremity,
It asked a Crumb - of me.

Once you've finished rearranging your altar, making it fit the you that you are today, spend a little time with it. Sit in front of it, perhaps meditate before it. Allow its magic and energy to support you.

Aromatherapy Practice

For a peaceful blend of essential oils that will soothe the mind and enchant the senses, choose from the following:

TOP NOTES

✳ MYRTLE. A soft, fresh, sweet scent, less citrusy than most top notes. Its gentle qualities help you to feel relaxed and held safely.

✳ SWEET ORANGE. This warm, sweet scent is simply happy. It's bright and optimistic, and yet kind—it doesn't ask you to go out and do anything, but just to sit and enjoy.

✳ ROSALINA. Soft and floral, with a slight medicinal bite. For when you need an extra breath of fresh air.

✳ YUZU. This citrusy scent calls for new beginnings, for a release of what's been bothering you.

MIDDLE NOTES

✳ CHAMOMILE. The most soothing of all scents, like a cup of tea made ephemeral.

✳ GERANIUM. Somehow both rosy and citrusy, this is a cheerful and uplifting scent.

✳ LAVENDER. The scent of lavender can calm the most active nervous system almost instantly.

✳ PALMAROSA. Lemony and woody with a slight hint of flowers. Provides emotional comfort.

✳ ROSE. Nothing supports the heart more than rose—this loving scent will carry you through.

BASE NOTES

✳ MYRRH. This spicy resin will unclog you, releasing tension and allowing for tranquility.

✳ PATCHOULI. Rich, earthy, and sweet, patchouli will help you relax, feeling warm and quiet.

✳ VETIVER. Deep and woody, this oil is often called "the oil of tranquility."

Once you've decided on your blend, create a mixture of one part base note, two parts middle note, and one part top note. You can use an essential oil diffuser or create a perfume oil by blending your essential oils with an unscented carrier oil like sweet almond or grapeseed oil.

Meditation Practice

In times of high stress, it's best not to try to get too fancy. This is not the time to learn a bunch of mantras or sutras or do any complex visualizations—if you're already anxious, that's probably only going to make things worse. Instead, start with something simple—indeed, sometimes that which appears the simplest contains the most powerful magic.

Get comfortable. If you have a zafu or zabuton to sit on, go for it, but the floor or a shady spot in the grass works just as well. You can light some incense or start a diffuser, or not. You can play some soothing music if you like or just listen to the birds or the sounds around you. Set a timer if you don't want to have to wonder how long you've been meditating, but you don't need to if you'd rather stay curious. Meditation requires nothing but your willingness and your breath.

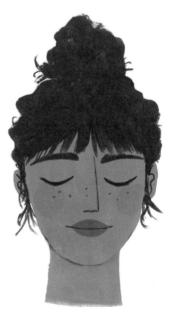

When you feel ready, close your eyes. Inhale for a count of six. Hold for a count of four. Exhale for a count of ten. Hold for a count of four.

Repeat this cycle, and once you've got the hang of it, bring in a simple visualization. On your inhale, imagine breathing in pure white light. As you hold, imagine that white light diffusing through your

36

body. As you exhale, imagine releasing anything that doesn't serve you—you don't need to focus on precisely what that might be, just imagine letting go of anything and everything. As you hold, feel the space you've created.

When your timer goes off, take a few moments to come back to your natural breath before you open your eyes. As you do so, feel that space, sense it expanding with light. Know that the light is always there for you.

Rune–Casting

Begin by holding your runes close to your heart as you ask them a question. When considering what the question could be, ask yourself—what is standing between you and a sense of peace and calm? Whatever comes to mind first is your answer. When you feel ready, reach into your bag and pull out a handful of stones. Don't try to pull out a specific number, as the runes you need are the ones that will find their way into your palm. Toss them gently onto your cloth.

Set aside any runes that have landed upside down with their carvings hidden from you, but leave the ones that are faceup in place, without touching them. Now, take your time. Observe how the runes relate to one another. Who is present? What do they have in common? What do they contradict? If two runes have fallen close together, you may want to consider combining their meanings, as they are likely intertwined. Or are they at war with one another? Rune-casting is simple to do, but interpreting the cast can be complex.

You can create a spread on your cloth to help guide the runes toward answering a more specific question, making them easier to interpret. You could mark three spots on your cloth, representing the past, present, and future, and then using the rune that landed closest to each spot to interpret your cast. As you and your runes get to know each other, you will devise ways to communicate with each other.

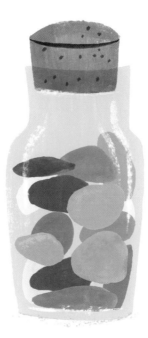

Feng Shui Support

If you're feeling uneasy or worried, you can adjust your surroundings to help you feel more at peace. Begin by inviting a little more of the earth element and the water element into your home. Earth will offer you a sense of being grounded and safe, while water will bring a mood of calm, of sanctuary.

If you've worked out a bagua system for your house, consider focusing on the self-knowledge or life purpose areas, as those are nourished by earth and water, but you should also take into account exactly what is stressing you out. If you're in a fight with friends, consider the friendship sector. Or if you're worried about work, maybe play around with the abundance sector, and so forth. You could also bring something that represents earth or water to the office, like a blue throw for those over-air-conditioned days or an earthenware coaster.

Now, you don't want to overdo it. Too much water can mean too much mystery, too much uncertainty, which can make you anxious, while too much earth can begin to feel smothering. Start small, adding just a bit

here and there. An indoor fountain is the most obvious and most powerful choice for calling upon the element of water, but it might also be a bit
too much. Start with perhaps a small mirror or a jar filled with pieces of
blue sea glass, and see where to go from there. For earth, a yellow or earth-
toned pottery vase is a good start or a square meditation pillow. It's easier
to add than subtract with interior decorating!

Spell to Banish Unwanted Thoughts

Our minds can be our own worst enemies. They can dwell on things we
cannot change, replay our worst moments over and over, and expend so
much energy on worst-case scenarios. They can overwhelm us with their
negativity.

But we are not our thoughts. They do not define us, and they certainly aren't always right. There are many things that we cannot change, but we *can* change our thoughts. This is something we have control over.

The first step is allowing those thoughts to exist. Just like with emotions, sometimes if we ignore a painful or troubling thought, it keeps coming back, until it starts yelling at us to pay attention and playing on a loop when we're trying to sleep. So go ahead and think it. You are thinking it anyway, after all. Take a piece of paper and write it down. It can be hard to look at, but remember, it's there anyway.

Is there something else? Write that down too. Keep going until you feel emptied of those thoughts—they are no longer in you; they are right there in front of you on the paper.

Now you have a few choices—this spell is for you to design. If it turns out those thoughts are something you want to keep close, if perhaps they are memories that are painful but still a part of you, you can paste them into a journal or place them inside a box of keepsakes. They can stay with you, but they don't need to be so present all the time.

But if these are thoughts that serve no purpose, that are only doing you harm, you can actually get rid of them. You can fold your piece of paper or even tear it into bits. You can give your thoughts over to the earth by literally burying them in the backyard. Or for a more dramatic statement, you can light them on fire and watch them burn to ash, transforming into a substance that nurtures the earth from which we came.

Once you've properly disposed of your thoughts, take a moment to reflect. The reality is that these thoughts aren't *gone*—it's not like you suddenly can't remember what they were. But you have taken a moment to really look at them and then given them the treatment they deserve. That is all they are worth, and you know that now.

Heart

Crystals for Peace

Because crystals are defined by their internal geometric patterns, you can enhance their effects by lining them up in a grid. By reflecting their internal geometric patterns in the external world, you can help bring your crystals into resonance with each other, allowing them to work together.

There are several different ways to create a crystal grid. If you're looking to invite peace, the more specific a structure you use, the better. Start by collecting a combination of the following crystals:

- Amethyst
- Apophyllite
- Clear quartz
- Moonstone

- Peridot
- Rose quartz
- Rutilated quartz
- Sapphire

- Selenite
- Sunstone
- Turquoise

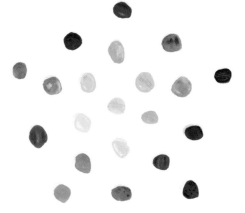

You'll want a total of eleven of these crystals, as follows:

✳ One center stone. Choose this stone carefully, as it will be the focus of your grid. What kind of peace are you looking for?

✳ Five stones for the internal ring. You can have five of the same kind, or three of one and two of another, alternating. Make sure these stones are approximately the same size and shape.

✳ Five stones for the middle ring. Again, you can have five of the same kind, or three of one and two of another, but either way make sure this group contains stones of approximately the same size and shape.

✳ For the external ring, you'll want to do something slightly different. Here, instead of choosing stones for peace, safeguard that energy by using stones of grounding and protection, including:

- *Black tourmaline*

- *Hematite*

- *Obsidian*

- *Smoky quartz*

You'll want five stones total, and again they can be a combination, as long as they are the same general size and shape.

Lay out your crystal grid as pictured, working from the center outward. Place your crystals carefully, keeping an equal distance between them. Remember, structure is important here. Once you've laid your final stone of the external ring, it is time to link the crystals. Take a quartz point or selenite wand, and working from the outside in, draw an invisible line connecting the outer stones to the middle ring, and to each other. Continue tracing the lines between the stones, connecting the middle stones to the inner ring, and finally to the center stone.

Leave your grid open for several days, running your fingers above it from time to time to feel its energy.

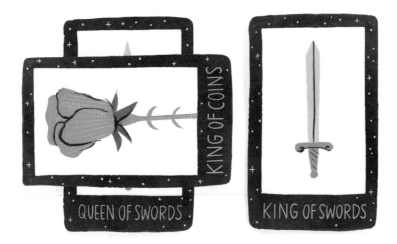

Tarot Reading to Find What to Let Go Of

This tarot spread is a simplified version of the classic Celtic Cross spread (see page 87). For now, you don't need to gain that level of insight from your tarot cards—this reading isn't about your life's purpose or an in-depth understanding of all you have going on in your life. Before you're ready to get into all that, you need to find a space of peace within yourself, to allow for all that uncovering. This spread will help you achieve that.

Begin by shuffling your cards. Take your time, and shuffle as long as you need to before you feel satisfied. Think of this as the time your cards need to listen to you, to hear what is going on in your world. Next, spread them out, laying them flat in a long line. Choose your first card and lay it in front of you. Choose your second card, and lay it across the first, perpendicular to it. Choose your third card, and place it to the right of the first two.

Your first card represents what you want, right now. Sit with it for a moment, before moving on to your second card. When doing a tarot reading, sometimes you'll feel an immediate agreement that this is indeed

43

what's going on for you. But there will also be times when the meaning of the card seems a little mysterious, and you're not quite certain how it applies. In many cases those are the times when we gain the most insight, so take a moment to come to terms with your first card.

Your second card represents what is crossing you at the moment— what is preventing you from getting what you want. Sit with this card, too. Often, it doesn't represent an enemy, or even anything particularly negative, and in fact it may even call into question whether the first card *is* what you truly want.

Your third card represents the way forward. It may suggest that there is a way to integrate the first and the second or that there is a third path open to you.

When you feel satisfied, close up your cards and put them away—but remember that you can always draw another card to ask for clarification. The cards are helpful like that.

You can allow the imagery of the cards to speak directly to you, or you can look to the symbolic meanings of suits and individual cards. For more detail on interpreting individual cards, see page 54.

Lunar Ritual

The moon is a powerful thing. It is a planet-shaped representation of feminine energy, with all the associated mystery. It invites us to use our intuition, our creativity, and our spirituality.

It can also be a pretty severe impediment to a good night's sleep. Its brightness can disrupt our circadian rhythms, and its pull—so profound that it can drag the waters of the tides for miles—can impact our hormones and our energy. All of that creativity, that intuition, that connection with mystery can keep us lying awake, wondering and worrying. This isn't very helpful, as a restless night tends to sap our energy, putting all of that

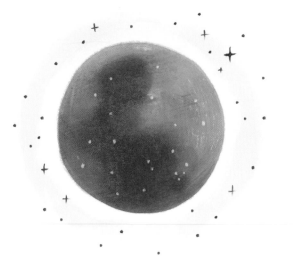

feminine creativity to waste. This ritual will help you channel the moon's energy, allowing you to sleep so that you can put it to good, productive use in the morning.

First, set yourself up for greatness. Get some window shades or an eye mask, and do all the things you know you need in order to have a good night's sleep: have an early dinner, and turn off your phone or television at least an hour before going to bed.

Spend that hour in quiet contemplation. Allow the moon its time with you. You can begin by making a cup of restful tea using vervain, valerian, lemon balm, chamomile, and betony. You'll only need a total of a teaspoon to brew a cup. If you can, sit in the moon's light as you sip your tea. Keep a journal handy, and write down any thoughts that come to you. Allow those thoughts to flow out of you onto the page—you won't need them overnight. They will keep until morning.

When you're ready for bed, set your journal next to you on the night-stand or someplace nearby. Lower your window shades or use your eye mask, and as you close your eyes, ask the moon to communicate to you through your dreams. When you wake up, write them down in your journal. If their meaning isn't immediately clear, don't worry. Your intuition will help you discover it.

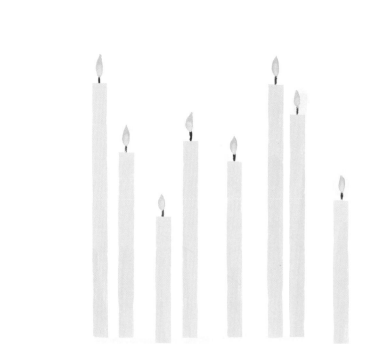

Candle Spell

The heart is the center of all our emotions. Just as our heart cannot stop beating—or it would be pretty terrible if it did, anyway—neither can we stop having emotions. They are always with us, and being "emotional" is not a bad thing—it is simply a state of being alive. So the idea behind feeling at peace is not feeling devoid of emotions, but about finding a way to be at ease with your emotions. If you're angry about something, then you're angry—that emotion isn't going to go away just because you want it to. But you can find a way to allow that anger to be felt and then to settle; it can recede, allowing you to be at peace with it—not despite it. This practice uses the power of candle magic to help you do that, so that you can live *with* your emotions and embrace them for what they have to teach you.

First, select your candle. Different candle colors have different meanings, and you should choose accordingly.

✳ WHITE. Dissipation of negative energy, peace, truth

✳ PURPLE. Intuition, peace, wisdom, healing

✳ BLUE. Meditation, healing, forgiveness, communication, happiness

✳ GREEN. Fertility, abundance, luck

✳ PINK. Friendship, harmony, joy, love

YELLOW. Confidence, creativity, clarity

✳ ORANGE. Energy, strength, courage

✳ RED. Passion, energy, vitality

Take a moment to select an anointing oil that will speak to your heart. You can use rose, vetiver, palmarosa, or myrtle essential oil or create a blend of your choosing. Anoint the candle with the oil, being careful to work on the edges of the candle and not touch the wick. If you like, you can also anoint your temples, the insides of your wrists, and the space above your heart.

Light the candle. As you gaze into the fire, watch how it flickers. Imagine the pulse of the flame coming into resonance with your heartbeat. And then, simply feel what you are feeling. If you are angry, be angry. If you are sad, allow that emotion to come through. Let the candle shine a light into your heart and allow your hidden emotions to reveal themselves.

And then, listen to them. What do they have to teach you? If you gain any insights, write them down in your journal. Once you've allowed yourself to hear what they have to say, give your emotions permission to settle. Gaze back into the flame, and imagine it burning through the feeling that you want to release. Imagine the intensity dissipating, like steam.

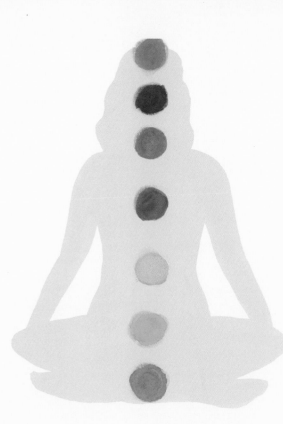

About Chakras

The word *chakra* can be a bit of a trigger—for a lot of people, it brings to mind the epitome of a modern hippie—which isn't at all a bad thing, but our impression of chakras is often that they're, well, imaginary.

In reality, chakras are just an ancient method of mapping the endocrine system, which is run by energy in the body—not calories or the stuff our mitochondria produce, mind you, but something more elemental, the kind of energy we experience throughout the universe. That energy is focused on seven specific areas of the body, and each of them is located along the spine. They are generally pictured as a wheel or a swirl—in fact, *chakra* in Sanskrit means "wheel."

Each chakra is connected by prana (also known as qi)—our essential life force—and each chakra has its own sound frequency as well as its own light frequency or color. Ideally, your chakras should all be open, spinning and churning, so that you can give and receive their energy. But from time to time, a chakra can become imbalanced, so that it is either overactive or blocked. A blocked chakra prevents your prana from moving through it, while an overactive chakra can dominate the others. In order for the body, mind, and spirit to be in tune—allowing you to live a harmonious life—your chakras need to be balanced. Each of them should have a free flow of energy moving both inward toward you and outward toward the world. When your chakras are in balance, you feel at ease within your whole self, as you are giving and receiving freely with the world.

THE CHAKRAS

MULADHARA. The root chakra is at the base of the spine, centered at the bladder and the colon. This is the most instinctual of all chakras—our fight-or-flight response is located here. This chakra governs our connection with our ancestors, our past, and our literal roots in the earth. Everything else stems from here, as the other six chakras cannot be fully functional unless we have the support of the root chakra. When the root chakra is blocked, we might experience leg and feet pain, as well as problems with the lower digestive tract. When we are feeling worried about our basic survival needs that might also indicate a blocked root chakra. On the other hand, when we are being irresponsible about money or our personal safety, then that means the root chakra is overactive—and we are not as safe as we think we are. When the root chakra is balanced, we feel, and are, utterly fearless and safe.

COLOR:	SOUND:	CRYSTALS:
red or black	LAM	obsidian, hematite, agate, bloodstone, bronzite, smoky quartz

SVADHISTHANA. The sacral chakra is just above the root chakra, where the ovaries and testes are—and you guessed it, this chakra governs our creativity and sexuality. Pleasure and passion, both physical and spiritual, stem from this chakra. When it's blocked, we are literally blocked. Writer's block, artist's block, an inability to be inspired or even to feel pleasure are all the result of a blocked sacral chakra. On the flip side, an overactive sacral chakra can provoke us to hedonistic or manic energies and behaviors. In either case, an imbalanced sacral chakra can cause physical problems like fertility issues, kidney trouble, or hip and lower back pain. But when the sacral chakra is balanced, we are more fertile in every way—we are sexually engaged and ripe with ideas and passions.

COLOR:	SOUND:	CRYSTALS:
orange	VAM	sunstone, rutilated quartz, carnelian, garnet, ruby, citrine

MANIPURA. The solar plexus chakra is beneath the breastbone, near the adrenal glands and the endocrine system. Manipura is about personal power, our sense of self and our inner strength. This is where we find the source of our willpower, the drive that takes us from inertia to action. A blocked solar plexus means that the critical inner voice we all have is constantly shouting at us. We might fear rejection and relegate ourselves to the sidelines of our own lives, while those with an overactive solar plexus chakra might be excessively dominating, overstressed, and may be in need of constant attention—someone who always demands the spotlight, whether it is positive or negative. Physical manifestations of imbalance include high blood pressure, chronic fatigue, and stomach ulcers. But a balanced solar plexus chakra gives us the confidence to make good choices in our lives. Someone with a balanced solar plexus chakra is assertive without being arrogant and in control without being afraid.

COLOR:	SOUND:	CRYSTALS:
yellow	RAM	tigereye, pyrite, yellow jasper, peridot, mookaite

ANAHATA. The heart chakra is, of course, at the heart, but also at the lungs. This central chakra is responsible for maintaining the balance between the other six. And how else is there to achieve that balance but with love and with the breath and space to allow those we love to be who they are and love us in return? This love includes romantic love, self-love, friendship, kindness, compassion, and respect. This is how we recognize that we are not alone, that we are part of a community, a partnership, a family. When the heart chakra is blocked, we cannot feel that love—we cannot allow it into ourselves, and we cannot demonstrate it to others. And when it is overactive, we become needy and can have difficulty setting healthy boundaries. This can show up physically as asthma or even heart disease, as well as shoulder and upper back pain. But a balanced heart chakra allows a life of love and support, with all the joy and space that brings.

COLOR:	SOUND:	CRYSTALS:
green or pink	YAM	rose quartz, morganite, malachite, emerald, rhodonite

VISUDDHA. The throat chakra is near the thyroid gland. If the first three chakras are internal and the heart is the balance, then the final three are about reaching outside of ourselves. The throat chakra is about speaking out, standing up for what we believe in, and showing up as our true selves with those around

51

us. When we are afraid to speak out or are presenting a version of ourselves to the world that isn't really true, then the throat chakra is blocked. On the other hand, if we are shouting at the world and speaking without compassion or interest in others, then the throat chakra is overactive. This can manifest physically in a hyperactive or hypoactive thyroid, a sore throat, neck pain, and mouth ulcers. A balanced throat chakra means that we not only speak the truth, but we can hear and accept it as well, as we live authentically in and with the world.

COLOR:	SOUND:	CRYSTALS:
light blue	HAM	aquamarine, turquoise, sodalite, blue lace agate

AJNA. The third eye chakra is near the pituitary gland. That third eye is a way of seeing things clearly. It's about observation and perception, but also wisdom—not just seeing, but seeing with truth and intuition. A blocked third eye cuts us off from the world around us, so that we look only within ourselves until we become paranoid and depressed. But an overactive third eye can result in too much examination of the world outside, so that we imagine things about others that simply aren't true and we become unfocused. Physical symptoms can include headaches, hearing loss, and blurred vision. But when the third eye chakra is balanced, we not only see what is happening around us, we comprehend it, feeling it deeply with compassion and understanding.

COLOR:	SOUND:	CRYSTALS:
indigo	OHM	lapis lazuli, azurite, fluorite, fuchsite, lepidolite, sapphire, labradorite, apophyllite

SAHASRARA. The crown chakra is at the very top of the head near the pineal gland and, of course, the brain. This chakra allows us to leave the self behind entirely, though of course it remains rooted in the other six chakras. Here we focus not just on what is outside the self, but what is *beyond* the self, beyond even the conception of self as it separates us from those around us—and from the spiritual world. Sahasrara connects us with all life and with the magical power of the spirit and the universe. When the crown chakra is blocked, we are isolated and lonely, bitter, and weighted by the difficulties of life, and when it is overactive, we can become arrogant, believing we know more than we do and holding ourselves separate and above those around us. Nightmares, migraines, and insomnia are the physical manifestations of this imbalance. But a balanced crown chakra allows us to find the best version of ourselves, that version that is tapped into the energy of all life.

COLOR:	SOUND:	CRYSTALS:
purple	OHM	sugilite, opal, amethyst, kyanite, clear quartz, celestite, apophyllite

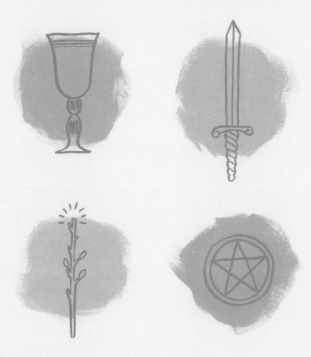

About Tarot

There's nothing truly magical about tarot. These cards were originally used for games . . . just like the playing cards we use today. And like playing cards, as physical objects they are really nothing more than pieces of paper with pretty pictures on them. They too have an arrangement from ace through ten, as well as four face cards—the page, the knight, the queen, and the king. Instead of hearts, spades, diamonds, and clubs, the suits are Cups, Pentacles, Swords, and Wands, and cards within these suits are known as the Minor Arcana. But a tarot deck has an additional twenty-two cards, which are known as the Major Arcana. They move in a cycle, beginning with the Fool, passing through Death and the Tower—which don't mean quite what you think they do—and ending with the World—a card of fulfillment.

If they're just pieces of paper, what's the point? They don't really tell the future, so what kind of divination is this? The thing about tarot is that it's at heart a sort of *internal* divination. It helps you see the answers *you already know* deep down. The cards can provide both confirmation for what we feel is right and a way to look at some hard truths—tapping into our essential knowledge, as if by magic. You'll find that every reading has something accurate to say, giving you a little chuckle or nod as you recognize it. Sometimes a reading knocks you flat out with something obvious you should have seen but were hiding from yourself. Most often what you feel is a sense of *relief*, knowing that what you thought was going on isn't just in your head. The cards help you trust your instincts, call you out on your hopes and fears, and best of all, point you in a direction for action. What do you want to do? What should you do? Are they the same thing or not?

The cards will never tell you anything you don't already know. You are giving your energy to the cards, and they are merely reflecting it back to you. Remember, they're just pieces of paper with pictures on them. As with so much magic, any power they have comes from what you bring to them.

You don't need any special training or to be an expert to do a tarot reading. It can feel like a lot of memorization, but you can start by looking up the meanings of each card—tarot decks always come with a book explaining the meanings. Still, as you work with the cards, you'll get to know your deck and how it speaks to you so that over time each card will have a meaning that is slightly different from what's in the book—it will be honed, narrowed, and specific to you and your associations. Because of this, you need to start by choosing a deck that provokes those kinds of associations. And there are *a lot* of decks to choose from. The traditional Rider-Waite and Aleister Crowley Thoth are the most common, but that doesn't mean that they will be the best for you. Look for a deck that attracts you, that is evocative, that makes you *want* to do a reading. A deck that you like is one that will respond to you, one that will speak to you.

Interpreting tarot requires balancing knowledge and intuition; the archetypes in each card provide history and grounding to your reading, but your own personal history will add detail and color to those archetypes, allowing you to see deeper and further.

THE SUITS

CUPS

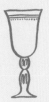

Cups are the suit of relationships. It's about our connections with those around us, and it's also about our feelings about those relationships. Cups are dominated by emotion, and choices made under the influence of Cups will be made with the heart, rather than the mind. This can be good or bad, depending on the situation. Most of the time, our hearts lead us true, but if you are driven *only* by your emotions, reason can be left by the wayside for some unrealistic expectations of those around you.

I **ACE.** Love, new relationships, beginnings

II **TWO.** Unity, attraction, intimacy

III **THREE.** Friendship, celebration, cooperation

IV **FOUR.** Apathy, contemplation, self-absorption

V **FIVE.** Regret, grief, failure

VI **SIX.** Nostalgia, childhood memories, innocence

VII **SEVEN.** Opportunities, choices, temptation

VIII **EIGHT.** Dissatisfaction, escapism, disappointment

IX **NINE.** Bliss, fulfillment, satisfaction

X **TEN.** Harmony, familial happiness, healthy relationships

P **PAGE.** Emotions, childlike curiosity, potential

KN **KNIGHT.** Romance, whimsy, fantasy

Q **QUEEN.** Intuition, nurture, in the flow

K **KING.** Emotionally mature, balance of logic and emotion, advisor

PENTACLES

 The suit of Pentacles—also known as Coins or Disks—is the suit of work and prosperity. How you define that work depends on who the reading is for—this could be a job, or it could be the work we do around the home, maintaining our family and relationships. It depends on the context, but, generally speaking, Pentacles refer to work for monetary gain because this suit is about practicality. It's about our most basic needs and goals—things we often consider less important than lofty ideas like creativity and relationships. They aren't, of course—without Pentacles, we wouldn't have the support or strength for anything else.

That said, if you are overly focused on Pentacles, you may lose sight of what's really important to you, on a soul level.

I **ACE**. New career opportunity, potential, abundance

II **TWO**. Ability to prioritize, adaptability, efficiency

III **THREE**. Collaboration, moving forward, organization

IV **FOUR**. Frugality, scarcity, overvaluing the material

V **FIVE**. Poverty, worry, isolation

VI **SIX**. Generosity, charity, receiving

VII **SEVEN**. Perseverance, investment, assessment

VIII **EIGHT**. Labor, skill development, hard work over time

IX **NINE**. Abundance, success, self-sufficiency

X **TEN**. Wealth, long-term stability, legacy

P **PAGE**. Learning a new skill, capability, motivation

KN **KNIGHT**. Productivity, hard work, focus

Q **QUEEN**. Working parent, nurturing, practical

K **KING**. Business, leadership, confidence

SWORDS

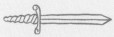 As you might guess, Swords are about conflict—something we all experience from time to time. And while these obviously aren't literal swords, they do cut with the clean sharpness of logic and intellect. The conflict here comes when the mind is battling with the heart. The instinct can be to turn away from Swords, to run from it, but just like with Pentacles, there is value here. Seeing things clearly, with logic and justice, is a necessity. Our hearts sometimes view only what we desire—not what's truly there. Swords reveal the facts, cold as they may be.

I **ACE.** Clarity, new ideas, breakthrough

II **TWO.** Difficult decision, stalemate, avoidance

III **THREE.** Heartbreak, despair, pain

IV **FOUR.** Rest, recovery, seclusion

V **FIVE.** Conflict, defeat, bad blood

VI **SIX.** Transition, letting go, change

VII **SEVEN.** Strategy, manipulation, betrayal

VIII **EIGHT.** Self-doubt, lack of choice, limiting beliefs

IX **NINE.** Anxiety, fear, depression

X **TEN.** Ordeal, tragedy, crisis

P **PAGE.** Seeking, desire for knowledge, new perspectives

KN **KNIGHT.** Ambitious, assertive lack of forethought

Q **QUEEN.** Hard truths, unsentimental, clear boundaries

K **KING.** Intellectual authority, power, advisor

WANDS

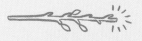

Wands are about striking a spark and allowing it to burn into the fires of creativity. They are primal energy, intuition, expansion, and actualization. They demand that you bring your true self out into the open. There is an element of danger in that, and Wands should always be balanced with the other three suits, but a life without Wands is a life unlived. If you encounter a spread dominated by Wands, then that means it's time to pursue that creative dream. That may not necessarily mean taking a painting class or writing a novel—though it might! It might also indicate starting your own business, taking a risk, even having a child. Creation is as individual as each of us.

I **ACE.** Inspiration, creativity, enthusiasm

II **TWO.** Planning, goals, decisions

III **THREE.** Progress, sharing ideas, exploration

IV **FOUR.** Celebration, early success, small rest period

V **FIVE.** Opposition, roadblocks, conflicting opinions

VI **SIX.** Success, pride, self-confidence

VII **SEVEN.** Protection, perseverance, competition

VIII **EIGHT.** Action, fast pace, change

IX **NINE.** Resilience, capability, strength

X **TEN.** Responsibility, commitment, completion

P **PAGE.** Discovery, free spirit, curious

KN **KNIGHT.** Energy, passion, impulsivity

Q **QUEEN.** Power, determination, courage

K **KING.** Leadership, honor, vision

THE MAJOR ARCANA

O THE FOOL. Idealism, innocence, potential. The Fool can be both positive and negative, containing the innate wisdom of a child, but also the potential for naivety.

I THE MAGICIAN. Power, resourcefulness, achievement. This is a real magician—no parlor tricks here. This is someone skilled and capable, who can do just about anything they set their mind to.

II THE HIGH PRIESTESS. Unconscious, dreaming, mystical. The more feminine side of the Magician, more mysterious and intuitive. When she appears in a reading, she is asking you to see the unseeable inside yourself.

III THE EMPRESS. Earth Mother, creation, fertility. This sensuous, loving mother figure is a call to nurture and be nurtured, by the earth and by those who mean the most.

IV THE EMPEROR. Tradition, authority, rules. The quintessential leader, who is just and fair, though sometimes unable to see other points of view. Ask yourself whether you need more—or less—structure in your life.

V THE HIEROPHANT. Establishment, learning, conformity. This card represents an entire belief system, which could be religion, gender society, politics—it depends on the context in your life.

VI THE LOVERS. Duality, love, harmony. This card can mean a literal romantic relationship or an easy, peaceful marriage of two disparate parts within yourself.

VII THE CHARIOT. Balance, self-control, willpower. Sometimes those parts within us aren't so easy and peaceful. The Chariot is about the work in finding that balance.

VIII STRENGTH. Resilience, fortitude, self-confidence. This is about strength in the long term, to get through a difficult situation over time—and do it well.

IX THE HERMIT. Spirituality, solitude, wisdom. The introvert's favorite card. It asks you to take some time to contemplate, to step back from a situation so you can gain some clarity.

X WHEEL OF FORTUNE. Luck, destiny, cycles. This card asks you to believe in something more, that there is a force for good in the world, guiding you through good times and bad.

XI JUSTICE. Fairness, truth, karma. Following that force for good is a reckoning—you will get what's coming to you (good or bad) eventually and so will everyone else.

XII THE HANGED MAN. Surrender, self-awareness, knowledge. Sometimes, we must sacrifice for knowledge, for truth. We must work for it, but the answers are there.

XIII DEATH. Change, transformation, endings. This is not literal death, but instead the death of a way of being. Perhaps it's a sign that you're about to start a new job or find a new way of relating to a family member.

XIV TEMPERANCE. Moderation, compromise, self-control. When this card comes up, it's a sign that you shouldn't rush into anything. Take a moment to listen to what others have to say and think things through.

XV THE DEVIL. Self-deception, the monster within, ignorance. You are always your own worst enemy. When the Devil appears, he is trying to tell you that the thing that is always getting in your way is showing up again.

XVI THE TOWER. Destruction, revelation, starting over. If Death is about change, the Tower is about starting over completely, but on the other side of this painful change you'll find peace.

XVII **THE STAR.** Hope, inspiration, spirituality. This is about new beginnings. Think of a star born of a nebula formed by a collapsed star, renewing again and again.

XVIII **THE MOON.** Illusion, subconscious, fear. In the moonlight, things can look unreal, and therefore scary—but there really isn't anything to fear. Use this time of unreality to explore what's possible.

XIX **THE SUN.** Clarity, confidence, positivity. Now you can see what's really going on and feel sure about your path.

XX **JUDGMENT.** Looking back, absolution, rebirth. Have you made good choices? Now is the time to evaluate—should you choose differently? The choice is always there to make and make again.

XXI **THE WORLD.** Completion, fulfillment, moving on. When this card appears, it is telling you that you have done what you wanted to do or you soon will if you follow the path.

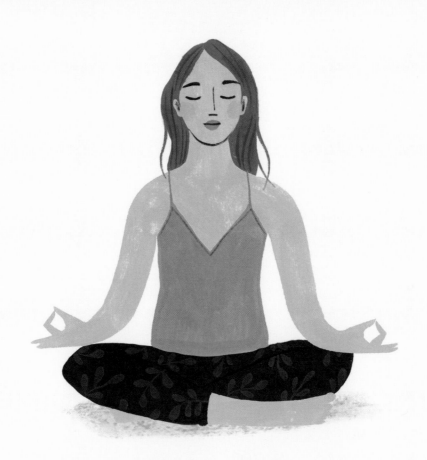

About Yoga

Yoga can be as simple as an exercise class or as complicated as a way of life. It is completely possible to attend a Power Yoga class, get a great workout, and leave it at that—but you can also go deeper. In Sanskrit, the word *yoga* means "union," as in the connection of the human with the divine. This understanding dates back 2,500 years, and if you were to google "yoga is" today, you would get thousands of different answers. (A personal favorite: "yoga is the goal of yoga practice.")

Widely regarded as the first known compilation of yogic philosophies, *The Yoga Sutras of Patanjali* was written sometime between 325 and 425 CE. They lay out *ashtanga*, a structure of the eight different limbs of yoga:

✳ **YAMA.** These are the first of the ten yoga ethics, beginning with the five "abstentions," things that a practitioner of yoga should engage in and never stray from: *Ahimsa*, to avoid violence toward any living being—essentially, do no harm. *Satya*, to avoid lies. We tend to find ourselves being, well, less than truthful in so many situations, often simply because it's easier or because we don't want to do the work that truth requires. *Asteya*, to avoid theft. This goes beyond simply not shoplifting and into carrying your own weight in the world and contributing to your community. *Brachmacharya*, to avoid faithlessness. This is often inflated to mean chastity, but at heart it's about viewing sex as a way of honoring yourself and those you love. *Aparigraha*, to avoid greed and embrace generosity. This is generosity of spirit as well as of wallet.

✳ **NIYAMA.** These are the second half of the ten yoga ethics, known as the "observances," or ways of life that a practitioner of yoga should always strive for: *Śauca*, purity of mind, speech, and body—essentially, showing up as the best version of yourself. *Santosha*, contentment and acceptance; a way of accepting reality as it is and finding peace and happiness with it, even as you work to make the world a better place. *Tapas*, perseverance. This is where that work comes in, as you put in the effort needed. *Svādhyāya*, reflection and study, as you seek the truth of who you are. Know thyself. *Ishvara pranidhana*, contemplation of the divine. This is the exploration of something more, of a force for good in the world.

✳ **ASANA.** In Patanjali's *Sutras*, this refers to the seated position used for meditation (now known as *sukhasana*), but is often used to define the different poses in a physical yoga practice. The goal here is both steadiness and comfort, so that you are sitting—or downward dogging—in such a way that you are both firm in strength, but also at ease in that strength. Most yoga we practice today is hatha yoga, which translates to "sun-moon." It's about finding the balance between force and rest. In practice, this means that you should never push your body into a twisted, uncomfortable position that it isn't ready for! Find a version of the pose that allows you to feel that balance.

✳ **PRANAYAMA.** Translating to "stretched breath," these are breathing exercises, often used in conjunction with asanas. *Prana* is often used to mean "life force," and *yama*, which we have already encountered, means "control." We have the ability to raise or lower our own heart rates and to intentionally harness our own breath—both of which, together, serve our life force. Pranayama focuses on the inhalation, the exhalation, and the space between.

✳ **PRATYAHARA.** This translates to "abstraction" and is the first of the internal stages of yoga, according to Patanjani. Here, the practitioner brings some distance between their internal world and the external world, moving away from their five senses—taste, touch, smell, hearing, and sight. You know when you're reading a great book, and you're so involved in it that you don't notice any disturbances? They're there, and you hear them, but you're simply not bothered by them? Pratyahara is that feeling of not being bothered—though it would happen free of the distraction/pleasure of a good book.

✳ **DHARANA.** *Dharana* means "concentration." The idea here is to build on pratyahara and find a single point of focus. When mindfulness meditation practices encourage you to focus on your breathing, this is a form of dharana. Reciting a mantra over and over, chanting, or even gazing at a single spot of focus—as in a candle spell, for instance—are all forms of dharana.

✳ **DHYANA.** Building even further, dhyana brings us to meditation. This can mean a sustained form of dharana, or it can mean a deep contemplation of the self or any other object of focus. There is intention here; rather than simply focusing, you are going deeper into finding meaning or truth. And yet, as in hatha yoga, you are seeking the balance between force and rest—you have intention, but you are not actively searching. Instead, you are receiving.

✳ **SAMADHI.** When you move beyond meditation into a trance state, you have reached samadhi. Yogananda, an influential guru in the 1920s, defined it as "a blissful super consciousness state in which a yogi perceives the identity of the individualized soul and the cosmic spirit." It is, essentially, enlightenment.

Samadhi is not a goal in this book, and you certainly won't be asked to go vegan or swear to tell the truth, the whole truth, and nothing but the truth. But to throw another "yoga is" in the mix, yoga is the *pursuit* of yoga, just as magic is often the *pursuit* of the magical. It's all a journey, and it can be no more and no less than what you make of it. The ethics of yama and niyama do provide a pretty good framework for a way of life, and the internal stages of pratyahara, dharana, dhyana, and even samadhi all fall under the umbrella of what today we call simply "meditation." If you want to tighten that booty and work off a little stress with some yoga, then roll out that mat—you'll be more flexible, stronger, and have better posture and balance. If you want to throw in some breath work to support your stretches and strength training, even better, as it will give you more energy, lower your blood pressure, and help you relax. If you want to add in some meditation, then, according to science, you'll experience reduced stress and anxiety, improvements in mood and optimism, greater self-awareness, greater attention span, reduced memory loss, and better sleep. And if you do all of that and live life like a good human, you're following Patanjali's eight limbs of yoga.

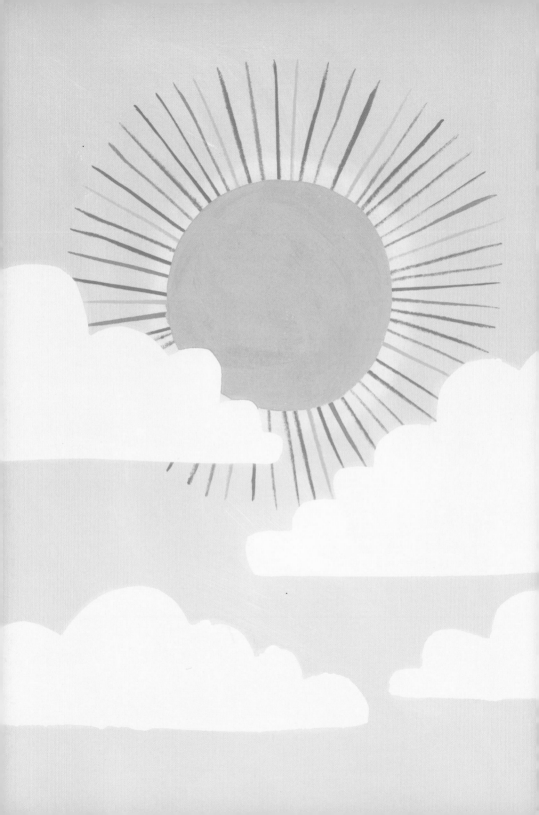

CLARITY

the quality of being coherent and intelligible—or the quality of transparency or purity

WE ARE SOMETIMES UNINTELLIGIBLE, EVEN TO OURSELVES. *What do I really want? What do I really mean? How do I really feel?* These questions sometimes seem impossible to answer, though as both philosophy and magic teach us, we are the only ones who can. When we look inside, we feel opaque.

This is partly because of all the distractions, all those disturbances that prevent us from being at peace—with ourselves and the world around us. When we are stressed, it is hard to think clearly. It's too much effort to answer these questions, to search for clarity. We're exhausted all the time.

But once you've found a general stasis within yourself, an inner calm, you'll begin to see the fog lift. You'll find the space and ease that will allow you to put that effort in. You'll begin to find that transparency, that purity of thought, and you will begin to know yourself.

Body

Clarity Tea

This tea will help lift the fog. It will allow you to look deep inside yourself and see your own desires and emotions clearly. It is best consumed at night, ideally under a full moon, so that its intuition-sparking light can aid you in your inner explorations.

Mix one teaspoon's worth of some combination of yarrow, wormwood, rosemary, marigold, and lavender. Pour some just-boiled water over it and allow it to steep for five minutes. Let the brew rest in the moonlight until it is cool enough to drink. Watch the steam floating through the light. If you like, play with it a little, twirling your fingers through it. Inhale its scent.

When it's cool enough, sip your tea slowly. Ask yourself the questions you most want answers to, queries that no one but you could ever answer. *What do I want? What is the right choice? What do I have to offer the world? What makes me happy?* Don't look at your phone. Don't read. Don't chat with others. Just sit and drink. If thoughts come to you, write them down in a journal. The answers are inside you—all you have to do is look.

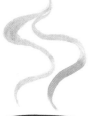
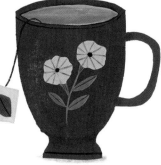

Throat Chakra Practice

Clarity works both ways. We can get clear inside ourselves on what we believe and what we want, but if we can't communicate it to others, then it doesn't do us a whole lot of good. No matter how open your third eye chakra is, if visuddha, the throat chakra, is closed, then you won't be able to speak your insights to others. This practice will stimulate the throat chakra, helping you to find your voice.

As with the other chakra practices, it involves chanting, which you may find uncomfortable, particularly if your throat chakra is indeed blocked. Lean into that discomfort and chant more loudly than perhaps you otherwise would. Push yourself to the edge of feeling a bit self-conscious, and make sure you give yourself the space and privacy to be vocal without the added awkwardness of someone listening in. If it feels weird and you wonder if you're doing it right, don't worry. You are.

Gather a crystal related to the throat chakra—aquamarine, turquoise, sodalite, or blue lace agate. Sit comfortably on the floor or on a cushion, holding the crystal in your palm. It doesn't matter *how* you sit, as long as your spine is straight and you are in no danger of falling asleep. Begin by gently rocking your right ear to your right shoulder. Hold it there for a breath, then draw your left ear toward your left shoulder. Hold for a breath. Then draw your chin to your chest, and breathe, stretching the back of your neck. Lift your chin to the sky, exposing the length of your throat to the sky. Breathe.

Move into some gentle neck rolls, drawing a circle with your nose clockwise. As you do so, visualize the spinning chakra at the base of your throat turning with you. When you feel satisfied, place the crystal in the hollow at the base of your throat, holding it there gently with your hand. Close your eyes and breathe, focusing on the feeling of the crystal against your skin. Breathe and focus on nothing else until it no longer feels cool, but has come into harmony with your body's temperature.

71

Lower your hand, keeping the crystal cupped lightly in your palm. Continue to imagine that light blue swirl at the base of your throat. Take a deep breath in through the nose, and empty it out through the mouth. Take another deep breath, and as you release it, allow your breath to make a sound, drawing it out into a long, low syllable: HAM. "Huuuuuuuuum."

It may feel awkward and creaky at first, as if your voice hasn't been used in a while. Take another breath, and release it again: HAM. "Huuuuuuuuuum." Feel the vibration of the sound in your throat. Allow it to expand, until the vibration fills your entire body, resonating with the crystal in your palm.

Take a third breath: HAM. "Huuuuuuuuum." Feel that vibration begin to expand with the sound, until it fills the room and air around you.

Continue chanting for as long as it feels right. When you feel complete, breathe in deeply and release the breath in a silent sigh. The vibration, the communication you've achieved through chanting, is still there.

Take another deep breath in. Open your eyes up to the sky. Open your mouth and stick out your tongue to exhale in a lion's breath. Shake your head, releasing any tension the practice might have called forth. Give your crystal a squeeze in thanks, and as you go about your day, begin to explore what is different for you now. What truths can you speak? What space can you allow others? Observe.

Refreshing Facial Spray

This spray acts as a splash of water over the face, a burst of brightness to awaken dulled senses and spark your awareness. You can use it at the start of the day, during that midafternoon slump, or even right before an important phone call or meeting. It's also good for the skin, as this spray contains witch hazel, a natural astringent that reduces inflammation, prevents acne, and fights bacteria.

Start by collecting ¼ cup of some combination of the following herbs, fresh or dried:

- Caraway
- Mint
- Lemon balm
- Mugwort
- Rosemary
- Sage

Chop them up or bruise them in a mortar and pestle and then pour a quarter cup of boiling water over them. Allow the water to come to room temperature.

Strain out your herbs. Add your water to the following:

- ¼ cup alcohol-free witch hazel extract
- 15–30 drops of some combination of rosemary, mint, sage, or calendula essential oils

Pour your mixture into a glass spray bottle.

Energizing Yoga Practice

These yoga poses are designed to flow one into the next and then be repeated until the moves become fluid, almost like a dance. The instructions will guide you in how to move from one pose to the next. It might take a little bit to get comfortable, but eventually you will feel confident enough to repeat the flow at a decent pace, getting your heart pumping but not racing, your blood moving smoothly, and your body and mind filling with energy and motion.

HOVERING MARJARYASANA
(Hovering Cat)

Begin on your hands and knees in a tabletop position. Curl your toes under and then lift your knees so that they are hovering above the ground. Keep your spine straight, your gaze down at the ground, and your core engaged. Stay here for three breaths. Be strong and fierce.

ADHO MUKHA
(Downward-Facing Dog)

From hovering cat, without lowering your knees back to the earth, lift your hips up to the sky. Walk your hands forward until you feel comfortable, keeping the back straight and the heels reaching toward the earth. Lift your right leg to the sky, and then bend your knee and bringing it forward toward your heart, with your upper body in plank pose. Raise your right leg back up, and then bring it back to the chest, tightening your core. Repeat once more, then raise the right leg up to the sky before lowering it back to the ground in downward dog. Raise your left leg and bring it into your heart, repeating three times before raising your left leg up to the sky and lowering it back to the ground.

VASISTHASANA
(Side Plank)

Roll up and over, as though there were an invisible mountain beneath your hips, and come into plank pose. Turn to the side so that the outside edge of your right foot is touching the earth, with your left foot resting on top. Your right hand supports your upper body weight. Draw a line with your left hand up to the sky and take a breath. As you exhale, come back into plank and roll over to the other side, turning so that the outside edge of your left foot is touching the earth, with your right foot resting on top. With your left

HOVERING MARJARYASANA

ADHO MUKHA

VASISTHASANA

BHUJANGASANA

UTTHITA BALASANA

hand supporting you, draw a line with your right hand up to the sky and take a breath. Exhale and roll back to the other side. Repeat until you've done a total of three on each side.

BHUJANGASANA
(Cobra)

From plank pose, bend your elbows and lower down to the earth. Arch your back and raise your chest and gaze up to the sky. Inhale. Exhale and lower back to the earth. Inhale and arch up, and exhale as you return. Repeat once more, for a total of three.

UTTHITA BALASANA
(Extended Child's Pose)

From your belly, push yourself back. Spread your knees wide and sink your hips onto your heels, keeping your arms stretched forward. Roll your forehead against the earth and take three deep breaths. Raise your hips and press yourself back up to tabletop position.

Third Eye Chakra Practice

Ajna, the third eye chakra, is our connection to our intuition. It is the window through which we can see into ourselves and out in the world, unfiltered by all that clouds our vision. To open this window, begin by choosing a crystal. Lapis lazuli, azurite, fluorite, fuchsite, lepidolite, sapphire, labradorite, and apophyllite are all good options; take a moment and select the one that feels right for you today—connect to your intuition. Consider its color and its texture as well as its meaning. You'll want something small with a fairly flat, smooth edge.

For this practice, find a place where you can lie down flat. Choose a spot that is clean and as free of distractions as possible, while also not likely to make you want to fall asleep. A blanket spread under a tree would be great, while an unmade bed piled with laundry would be less so.

Begin in a comfortable seat, with your crystal close by. Place your hands together in prayer and begin to rub them together, fast and furiously. Cultivate some heat and energy here. Keep going, and then bring your hands, still in prayer, up to your third eye. Close your eyes and feel that heat move from your palms into your third eye. Inhale, and as you exhale chant OHM, "ohhhhhhhhm."

Without opening your eyes, relax onto your back. If you need to open your eyes to find your crystal, do so, otherwise just lift it up and place it on your third eye. Draw small clockwise circles with it, stimulating the chakra and following its movement. Inhale, and as you exhale chant OHM, "ohhhhhhhhhm."

Let the crystal rest on your forehead and allow your hands to rest at your sides or on your belly. Imagine a slight pulsing sensation, and feel that rotation of the chakra that you've stimulated—it continues even as your hands and crystal are at rest. Inhale once more, and chant OHM, "ohhhhhhhhm."

Allow your breath to relax, to fall into its natural rhythm. Rest there for a few moments, and when you're ready, remove the crystal and roll up to a seat. Keep your eyes closed, and bring your hands back to prayer, back up to your third eye. Take one last deep breath, and exhale quietly as you open your eyes.

Mind

Altar Practice

Begin by tidying and dusting your altar. When it's neat and clean, take a moment to survey it. What no longer applies to your needs in this moment? Is there a talisman meant to represent a desire or wish that has already been fulfilled or has changed? Or is there even just something that doesn't really speak to you right now? Remove anything that doesn't feel absolutely necessary. Altars tend to get cluttered—it's their nature—but from time to time you need to strip them back down to their basics.

You may want to leave your altar as is for the time being. But if you would like to actively invoke a sense of clarity, consider changing out your centerpiece for an incense burner and lighting some cardamom, lemongrass, or angelica incense. You might use celestite, clear quartz, lapis lazuli, or labradorite as a centerpiece instead, or you can light a smudge stick and leave it to smolder in a dish or abalone shell.

Finally, take a scrap of paper and rest it on your altar, open and blank. Every morning, take a moment to write something on this—just a word or a phrase, whatever comes to your mind. It can be nonsense or a fragment of a dream. Just pause and do this every morning for a full moon cycle. When the month is up, look at your paper again. Circle common themes and images. Write in your journal about what you have learned.

Aromatherapy Practice

For a blend that invokes clear sight and understanding, choose from the following:

TOP NOTES

✳ BASIL. This bright, sharp scent invites a clear, relaxed focus.

✳ FRANKINCENSE. This time-honored mystical resin has a slight balsamic scent and has been used for prayers, meditation, and rituals for thousands of years.

✳ LIME. This sparkly, zesty aroma awakens your senses, giving you a radiant energy.

✳ ROSEMARY. An herb of remembrance, rosemary provides you with focus and mental clarity.

MIDDLE NOTES

✳ BLACK SPRUCE. This warm yet piney scent gives a vibrant sense of support; it has a gentle and long-lasting energy rather than a bright flare.

✳ GINGER. Ginger, on the other hand, offers a burst of energy, waking up the senses with a sharp focus.

✳ PEPPERMINT. This clear-eyed scent is another big wake-up call.

✳ SARO. Herby and medicinal, this bright aroma has an uplifting warmth.

BASE NOTES

✳ OPOPANAX. This sweet resin is frequently used in meditation, rituals, and other forms of contemplation. It helps you feel grounded but present.

✳ PALO SANTO. This woody, smoky scent is wonderful at clearing

energies, allowing you to center yourself and focus your mind.

✳ YLANG-YLANG. Rich and exotic, this intense aroma creates harmony throughout the body, mind, and heart.

Create your blend with one part base note, two parts middle note, and one part top note. You can make a perfume oil by adding this mix to an unscented carrier oil like sweet almond or grapeseed or simply put it in an essential oil diffuser.

Meditation Practice

There's a bit of irony when it comes to meditation: thinking about nothing can help you think more clearly. Of course, it's impossible to *actually* think about nothing. Our brains don't exactly come with an off switch. Meditation is not really the act of thinking about nothing; instead it's a way of training your brain to focus on something very specific so that perhaps all those thoughts become a little less important and a little less front and center for a while.

It gets easier with practice, and the easiest place to begin is with the breath. Start by cultivating an audible breath, something you can hear. Ujjayi Pranayama, or "Ocean Breath," is a technique that helps you keep your awareness on the present moment.

Find a comfortable seat, either sitting cross-legged or on a chair. Make an effort to sit upright with your back straight. This will feel tiring at first, but again, it gets easier with practice and engaging your core will keep your back from getting sore. Inhale, and then exhale through the mouth as though you're trying to fog a mirror. Do you hear that sound? Do you feel that slight constriction in the back of the throat? Do this a few times more until it feels familiar. Now, try to find the same sensation on the inhale. Repeat until it feels comfortable. Finally, close your mouth and breathe through your nose, but with that same constriction. That is the Ujjayi breath.

When you feel comfortable, close your eyes and settle into your meditation. You can set a timer if you like. Breathe in this fashion for long, slow breaths. Imagine your breath dropping down to the base of your spine, somersaulting there like a swimmer doing laps, and then rising back up and out with your exhale. Keep going.

When the thoughts come—and they will—don't get frustrated. Just give them a little mental wave, and let them go on their way. Return to your breath.

Rune–Casting

As runes are Nordic in origin, it is inevitable that they will be tied up with stories of Odin. This Norse god of war and wisdom—two things that may seem contradictory to the modern mind—sacrificed so much in his pursuit of knowledge: his eye and even his life as he stabbed himself with a spear and then hung upside down from a branch of Yggdrasil, the World Tree, for nine days without food or water. It was during those nine days that, according to legend, he found the runes, pulling them from the Well of Urd at the base of Yggdrasil. With the runes, Odin was able to heal, bind his enemies and render their weapons worthless, put out fires, fight sorcerers, and even wake the dead.

So the story goes. Our ability to wake the dead or smother a flame with runes has, well, yet to be achieved, but we can use the runes to find answers. This layout, known as Odin's Nine, is particularly useful for the way it allows you to look at the entirety of a situation from all perspectives.

Runes one through six represent Odin's body, with one and five serving as his feet, three as his trunk, two and six as his arms, and four as his head, hanging down toward the Well of Urd. Runes seven, eight, and nine serve as Odin's spear.

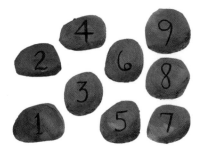

Approach this reading with a specific question in mind. And rather than scattering your runes as on page 37, reach into your bag and pull out runes one at a time without looking, much like when you pull tiles from a Scrabble bag. As you select each rune, lay them in numerical order, as they come.

✳ RUNE ONE. What has influenced you in the past around this question? What events have taken place?

✳ RUNE TWO. What is your present attitude toward those events and influences?

✳ RUNE THREE. What is influencing you now around this question?

✳ RUNE FOUR. What is your present attitude toward those influences?

✳ RUNE FIVE. What will stand in the way of your desired outcome?

✳ RUNE SIX. What do you really feel about that outcome?

✳ RUNE SEVEN. This rune represents the tools and skills you need—or already have—to combat or support runes one and two.

✳ RUNE EIGHT. This rune represents the tools and skills you need—or already have—to combat or support runes three and four.

✳ RUNE NINE. This rune represents the tools and skills you need—or already have—to combat or support runes five and six.

Feng Shui Support

In order to find clarity, you must start by clearing your space. Unfortunately, this means cleaning it. That's probably not what you want to hear, but it is necessary. Clutter, dust, messes untidied—all of these things nag at the backs of our minds, even when we think we're ignoring them. Work undone is a distraction, and in order to see past that distraction, you need to take care of it. So spend some time and go past the basics: don't just wash the dishes, do a full kitchen wipe-down. Don't just sweep the floors, mop them. Go through old magazines, clean out your closet, and take that pile of unwanted items to Goodwill.

When you're done, you'll be able to really see where you need to bring more clarity into your home. Start with taking away some of the element water. Water is soothing and wonderful for so many things, but in feng shui, clear it is not. Water is mysterious, unstructured, and unpredictable, and if you're looking for clarity, water may be a hindrance. Don't go overboard and take it *all* away, but remove a few objects that represent water for you, particularly in the bagua areas where you are most in need of some certainty.

Now it's time to add. Consider replacing those objects with things that represent metal. Metal is not water's opposite; rather, it is the structured, clear-eyed version. Consider that all metals can reach liquid form—so metal is essentially water made solid, made concrete and certain.

Remember, there can always be too much of a good thing. Too much certainty can make you blind to possibilities and to other points of view. Temper your metal with some fire—just a little. A splash of red or an occasional candle will do the trick.

Spell to Find Answers

Magic is a tool for discovery and can often lead to an increased understanding of ourselves and the world around us. Use this spell to uncover the answers to your own questions. Begin by creating a saltwater bath. Take a large bowl, big enough to cup your hands in, and fill it with very warm water. Dissolve half a cup of noniodized salt into it, stirring clockwise to harness the light of the sun. Sprinkle in some wormwood, sage, rosemary, mugwort, mint, lavender, caraway, or calendula—you can use whatever you have on hand. Allow your salt water to rest in the sunlight for at least an hour.

When you're ready, sit in the sunlight and splash your face with your prepared water. Smooth your hands across your forehead, your third eye, your temples, over your eyes, and down your throat. Repeat for a total of seven times. Do not dry off.

If you've made the perfume oil from page 79, use it to anoint your third eye. Close your eyes, and tilt your face up to the sun. Feel the air against your damp skin, and allow the warmth of the sun to evaporate the water. Feel that slight tightening as the salt dries. Inhale the scent of your perfume oil.

Now, ask the question: What is it that you most want to know? You may have begun this spell thinking of one thing but find now that your real question is something else. Don't seek the answer, just put the question out there. Imagine it flowing out of you through your third eye and dissolving into the air around you.

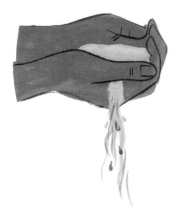

When you feel the question floating away, simply wait for an answer. Don't stretch for it, just keep your third eye open and receptive. Pay attention to what comes. It may come in the form of yet another question, or you may sense a deep certainty. When you feel the spell is complete, open your eyes. Take a moment and write down any insights you've received in your journal.

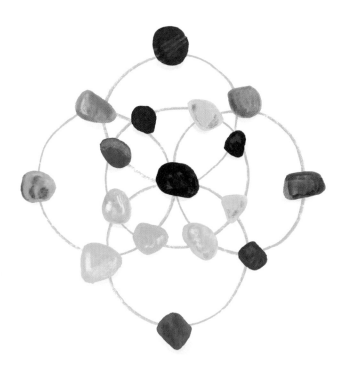

Heart

Crystal Grid for Focus

For this crystal grid, you'll want to be very precise. In order to really harness the focus-enhancing properties of these crystals, you want to make sure they are truly aligned geometrically. You may want to use a grid mat—you can purchase something or print one off of the internet, but it's also very simple to draw yourself, with a bit of patience. Take a large sheet of paper and use a ruler to pencil a straight line across the center. Rotate the paper ninety degrees and draw a second line perpendicular to the first through the center of the paper. Take a compass—remember those from elementary school?—and use it to draw a four-inch diameter circle right at the center of your line. Placing the point of your compass at the right edge of your circle, still on the line, draw another four-inch diameter circle. Now place the point of your compass at the left edge of your circle, still on the line, and draw a third four-inch diameter circle. Your three circles should overlap, with the edges of the outer circles touching each other at the center of the first. If you don't have a compass, you can also use the bottom of a glass. Rotate your paper ninety degrees and repeat the process, drawing two more circles around your original circle, for a total of five.

The spots where the circles intersect will be where you'll place your crystals.

You'll need a total of seventeen crystals. Place your largest stone at the center, and try to use evenly sized ones for the rest. You'll want to save four larger ones for the outside edges of the circles. Use a combination of the following stones:

o Apophyllite	o Clear quartz	o Peridot
o Aquamarine	o Fluorite	o Sapphire
o Azurite	o Howlite	o Selenite
o Blue lace agate	o Labradorite	o Sodalite
o Celestite	o Lapis lazuli	o Sunstone

Once you've placed your crystals on your grid, use a quartz point or selenite wand to draw energetic lines connecting each stone to the others. Leave your grid open for several days, ideally in a place where you work or study.

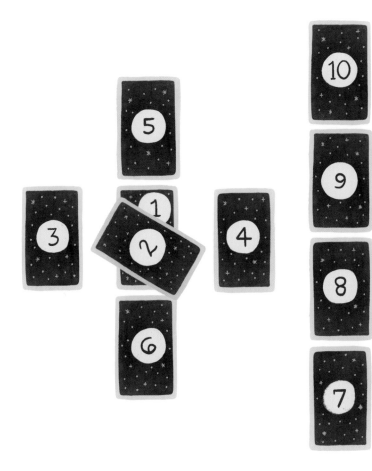

Celtic Cross Tarot Spread

The Celtic Cross is a classic tarot spread, and it has only gained in popularity in the many, many years it has been in use. That popularity is due to how very useful it is; the answers to any question, no matter how complex, can be found in this spread. Remember, nothing told to you here will be anything you don't already know, deep down.

1. This card represents you, how you are at this moment in time. What is going on with you? What are you experiencing, and how are you reacting to that experience?

2. Crossing the first card is the second; this card literally represents whatever is crossing you, whatever in your life is running antithetical to what you want and who you are.

3. What has happened in the past to create this situation?

4. This card represents the immediate future—it is not the resolution of the situation, but it can give you some idea of what will happen next.

5. What do you want? What are your goals? What do you believe is the right thing here?

6. The sixth card questions the answers given in the fifth. Perhaps that was only what you think you want or believe to be right. What does your intuition, your subconscious think? Are they in agreement?

7. What are your best next steps? This card will advise you.

8. The eighth card reminds you that you can only control what you do. There are external influences represented here, and they can have an impact on the situation, too.

9. This card speaks to your hopes and fears. it can often be difficult to interpret, since the two are frequently intertwined. Look back to the answers given in the sixth card, and see how the two relate.

10. The resolution. How will this situation play out? What will happen in the end? if the answer given by this card is not the one you want, know that you have the power to change it. if you keep on your current course, this is what will happen. This card will tell you if you need to take a different path.

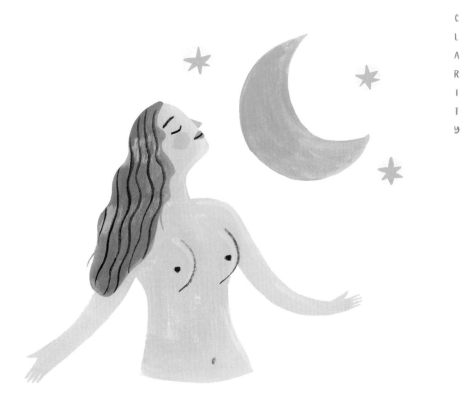

Lunar Ritual

Lunar rituals have been performed in countless cultures, likely beginning the very moment humans looked up at a clear night sky. And in almost every culture, the moon has been associated with the feminine and found representation in the form of a goddess. Artemis, Bendis, Gleti, Selene, Changxi, Ratih, and Hina are just a few of the different faces of moon goddesses throughout the world. But the moon goddess most associated with magic is Hecate. She ruled over herb lore (she taught Medea of Jason and the Argonauts fame everything she knew, though it is unknown whether Hecate approved of the use Medea made of her magic) and over the crossroads: as a liminal goddess, she managed the space "between," that place of almost, but not quite, a realm of imagination, possibility, and potential.

It is for this reason that she is associated with the moon, for the moon is both light and dark. Moonlight is full of nascent dreams crossing into reality, and this ritual is designed to aid in that transformation. It is best performed on the night of the full moon, when its crystalline light is at its brightest and most illuminating, in all senses of the word. If you can get outside and walk on the earth, you should do so, but a slant of moonlight from a window will do.

Wear a robe or something low-cut. There's no need to get naked here—though you certainly can if you want! Simply allow the light of the moon to fall directly on the skin over your heart. Feel its push and pull, and allow your heartbeat to come into resonance with that eternal rhythm. Inhale the moonlight and remember that even light is liminal, in the space between, as it functions as both a particle and a wave at the same time.

Do not force anything into or out of this space of possibility. Simply allow. If you want to, you can howl at the moon, or you can simply breathe a gentle sigh.

Candle Spell

Begin by selecting a white candle for purification and truth and a yellow candle for clarity. Arrange them side by side. Anoint the white candle with lavender or sage essential oils, and anoint the yellow candle with lemon balm, mint, or rosemary essential oils, being careful to stay well away from the wick. Create a blend of the oils you used and apply this to your temples and the soles of your feet.

When you're ready, light the white candle. Once the wax has begun to melt, carefully sprinkle some dried lavender or sage into the pool of wax, avoiding the flame. Light the yellow candle, and sprinkle some dried mint, lemon balm, or rosemary into its pool of wax, being careful to stay well away from the flame.

Inhale as you stare into the flames. As you exhale, close your eyes, and see the afterimage of the flames against your eyelids. Inhale and gaze upon the flames, exhale and gaze upon their echo. As you breathe in and out, consider the ways in which we look at and interpret the world every day. When we see a bee, we don't just see a bee; we see the potential of being stung and we see a manufacturer of honey. We see a creature the world depends on.

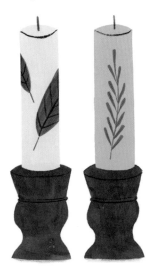

As you watch the flame flare and go dark as you open and close your eyes, meditate on how you constantly interpret and reinterpret your own life. As you do this, you will find that your eyes see both the flames and their afterimages at the same time—and that is where the truth lies. The world is always both what is and what we believe it to be at the same time.

What will you choose to believe?

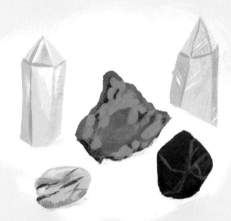

About Crystals

Crystals are formed when liquid matter cools and hardens in such a way that the molecules sort themselves into a repeating pattern—making what are essentially really pretty rocks!

But there's more to them than just looks. Unlike igneous or sedimentary rocks, crystals are formed over millions of years, and their slow, ancient growth helps us connect with the power of the earth. Those detailed geometric patterns create vibrations, as the molecules resonate within their formation. These vibrations are how crystals can store specific energies and information—which we can then use. Clear quartz, for instance, is employed in watches, memory chips, ultrasound devices, and more to store information like an unchanging time, a steady frequency, etc.

If a crystal can power a watch, what else can it do?

The reality is that people have been harnessing the practical and mystical powers of crystals for thousands of years. Through healing rituals, divination practices, burial rites, symbolization of power or meaning—think crowns studded with gems or even diamond rings—and protective spells, our ancestors incorporated crystals into the most profoundly important areas of their lives.

There are several different shapes of crystals, and each can be used in a different way:

WAND. Rough at one end and pointed at the other, these kinds of crystals are often used in jewelry or as protective amulets. They can also be applied to activate crystal grids, as this shape allows you to direct the crystal's energies in a more targeted way.

CHUNK. The larger crystals you see are often chunk crystals. They have essentially been mined and presented as is, so geodes, uncut turquoise, pyrite, etc., are considered chunk crystals. These larger ones release their energy in a more diffuse way, so they're good for general household use.

CUT. This is when a crystal or gem has been shaped to enhance sparkle and capture light, which amplifies the crystal's energies, making them even more powerful.

TUMBLED. These are the stones you'll find in bins at a science or mystical shop. They are smooth and shiny and comforting to hold.

TYPES OF CRYSTALS

One step into a mystical shop will tell you there are *a lot* of crystals out there. How do you choose? Each stone has a particular meaning/function that has been determined as it has been used throughout history. That's certainly helpful, but trust your instincts, too. When you're sifting through all those bins at the shop, you might find yourself drawn to a particular stone, so that the stone chooses you, rather than the other way around. That's worth paying attention to! What attracts you? Remember, the rocks are pretty, *and* they have meaning. What you find appealing on a purely visual level might be your mind telling you exactly what you need.

Pick up the stone that is calling you, and hold it in your hand. Does it feel warm or cool? Do you feel any vibrations or pulses? What is your emotional response to the stone? If you feel in resonance with the stone, then it is right for you.

It's possible, even likely, that from time to time you will need a combination of stones, such as obsidian, hematite, and pyrite for protection or amethyst and lapis lazuli for intuition. Experiment!

And if you're not sure, try clear quartz. It's the salt in the spice cabinet of crystals.

MOST COMMON STONES AND THEIR USES

AGATE. Invites courage, strength, and self-confidence.

AMAZONITE. Protects against electromagnetic stress and seasonal affective disorder, as well as encouraging self-determination and leadership abilities.

AMETHYST. Develops intuition and spiritual awareness. Aids in meditation, calm, and tranquility. Relieves headaches.

APOPHYLLITE. A calming stone that cleanses the third eye and crown chakras, releasing tension.

AQUAMARINE. Aids in expressing your personal truth. Reduces fear and tension.

AVENTURINE. This "stone of opportunity" invites luck and wealth.

AZURITE. Helps find spiritual or psychic blocks that are causing physical blocks. Transforms fear into understanding. Good for arthritis and joint pain.

BLACK TOURMALINE. A stone of protection. Places an energetic boundary between you and the energy of those around you.

BLOODSTONE. Helps you find your inner strength and tap into your courage and vitality.

BLUE LACE AGATE. This gentle stone of communication helps alleviate anger and tension.

BRONZITE. Energizes and protects, so that you have the strength and backup needed to tackle any challenges.

CALCITE. An energy amplifier, it eases communication between the physical and spiritual worlds.

CARNELIAN. Enhances creativity and sexuality and helps with exploring past-life experiences. Aids in digestion and soothes menstrual pain.

CELESTITE. Allows you to stand back and look at a problem without emotional clouding. Clears any blocks that may be preventing you from connecting with the spirit world.

CHRYSOCOLLA. Also known as the Goddess Stone, chrysocolla helps tap into feminine power.

CITRINE. A stone of abundance, invites success and money, raises self-esteem. Good for the heart, kidneys, liver, and muscles.

CLEAR QUARTZ. A stone of healing, channels power and amplifies universal energy. This stone can be programmed to whatever use you require.

DIAMOND. Symbolizes purity and innocence and encourages truth and trust.

EMERALD. The "stone of successful love," emerald encourages you to give and receive love.

FLUORITE. Useful in decision-making and helps with concentration.

GARNET. A stone of health and creativity, it stimulates your internal fire. Wards off cancer, good for skin elasticity, and also helps prevent nightmares.

HEMATITE. A stone of protection and grounding, it closes your aura to keep out negative energy. Provides support for astral projection.

HOWLITE. Eliminates anger, so that you can approach a situation with a calm heart and a clear mind.

IOLITE. Balances male and female energies and aids in self-acceptance.

JADE. Will inspire you to ambition and keep you working toward your objective. Good for longevity.

KYANITE. Kyanite can move energy through your body, calming you. It encourages communication and psychic ability.

LABRADORITE. Helps you see past any blocks or illusions to divine your true life's work.

LAPIS LAZULI. A stone of focus, helps amplify thought, aids in meditation, releases from melancholy. Good for sore throats and fever.

MALACHITE. Releases stored emotions, allows you to look inward. Useful in easing mental illness.

MERLINITE. A "stone of storms," merlinite can help those who have been hurt move forward in life.

MOOKAITE. A stone of adventure, mookaite will give you direction and a sense of the power of your own possibilities.

MOONSTONE. Soothes the emotions as well as the digestive system. Encourages peace and harmony within.

MORGANITE. A useful stone for teachers, morganite helps you to love without attachment.

OBSIDIAN. A stone of protection, particularly from spiritual forces. It will help you to understand and face your deepest fears. Helps with bacterial and viral invasions.

OPAL. Stone of amplification, enhances mystical experiences and creativity. Balances mood swings.

PERIDOT. Used since ancient times as a symbol of the sun, it invites energy, positivity, and light.

PYRITE. Stone of defense and protection, symbolizes the sun and cleanses the blood.

RHODOCHROSITE. A stone of self-love that helps to recover from emotional wounds.

RHODONITE. A stone of compassion, rhodonite can clear scars of the past and grow beyond them.

ROSE QUARTZ. A stone of love, not just romantic love, but familial and brotherly love, as well. Nurturing and comforting, this stone dissipates anger.

RUBY. The "stone of divine creativity," ruby inspires energy, passion, and power.

RUTILATED QUARTZ. This type of quartz is threaded with golden veins known as "angel threads" or "Venus hairs." It can aid in combating depression and can strengthen your will.

SAPPHIRE. A stone of wisdom that can ease depression, anxiety, and insomnia as well as heal eye and blood disorders.

SARDONYX. A stone of courage that can bring happiness and balance to romantic relationships.

SELENITE. A form of gypsum crystals often in wand shape, selenite is used for clearing and purifying negative energies and activating positive ones.

SHATTUCKITE. Aids in processing and understanding psychic experiences.

SMOKY QUARTZ. A stone of protection, it stimulates your survival instincts. Enhances focus and fertility.

SODALITE. A "stone of truth," sodalite will help you speak your own truth, as well as accept the truths of others, no matter how hard they may be to hear.

SUGILITE. This stone helps us engage with our intuition, with our spiritual awareness. It encourages positive thoughts, and can help you set aside sorrow and fear.

SUNSTONE. An antidepressant that stimulates the kidneys and allows energy to flow freely throughout the body.

TIGEREYE. A stone of stability, enhances personal power and integrity.

TURQUOISE. A stone of healing, guards against disease and environmental pollutants.

YELLOW JASPER. Stimulates the pancreas and the endocrine system, helps align the energy meridians.

HOW TO CLEAR AND ACTIVATE YOUR CRYSTAL

If your stone had been mined directly by your own hand, you would be good to go from here. But for most of us that isn't exactly a possibility! In all likelihood, your stone was found by others, packaged by others, handled by others, and it will have absorbed their energies.

Good or bad, you don't need that. This stone is *yours,* and you need to wash it clean. You can do this by soaking it in salt water or holding it under running water—preferably a stream, but rain or even your faucet will do in a pinch. Some of the flakier, lower on the Mohs scale of hardness stones are too delicate for that, though, in which case you can let them rest overnight—in the moonlight, if you can—next to carnelian or clear quartz, which have cleansing properties.

Once you've cleared your stone, it's time to activate it, enhancing the stone's inherent power by giving it an intention, pouring your energy, the vibrations of your specific needs into the stone. Clear quartz in particular can become whatever you need it to be and do whatever you need it to do. This is a very simple process. Just hold the crystal in your hand and think about your intention. The crystal will hear you.

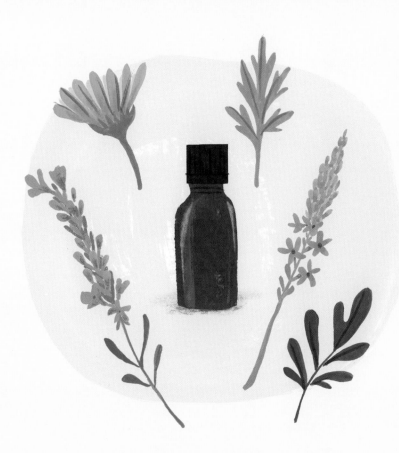

About Herb Magic

Herb magic can mean anything that utilizes the power of plants. In essence, chamomile tea is herb magic; it's an elixir of calmness. Hedge witches of old knew the secrets behind every possible plant, for every imaginable remedy, and their skills kept people alive in a time before modern medicine. So taking aspirin—which is derived from willow bark—for a headache or echinacea to ward off a cold is just the modern form of herbal healing.

But there's something so much more empowering—not to mention fun—about crafting your own herbal remedies rather than just popping a pill. Tending an herb garden, hanging them to dry, and making teas and tinctures are a way of making what is natural feel magical. The truth is, of course, that herbal healing *is* magical, regardless—for what could be more powerful than working with the earth and the life around us to enhance our own lives? But that connection, that interchange of energy, is removed when all we do is open a plastic bottle. In order to feel that connection, we must get closer to the source, as we used to be.

And herb magic doesn't have to just include things you consume. Lotions and balms made with all-natural ingredients are also good for your skin—perhaps even better—and to take all this magic a step further, you can use herbs in the same way you do crystals—to harness the energy of the earth with intention. Just as lavender has soothing properties that make us feel rested, so does mugwort help you feel more connected to the power of the universe. Placing specific plants around the home, consuming them, burning them, carrying them with you—these are all the most common and effective ways of bringing herb witchery into your life.

MOST COMMON HERBS AND THEIR USES

✳ **BETONY.** Useful in combating headache and insomnia, as well as warding off nightmares, it can also lower blood pressure. It is safe for consumption and can be used for purification and protection.

✳ **CALENDULA.** Also known as marigold, it grows easily and well and is also available dried. It is good for skin irritations, to calm an upset stomach, and is useful in divination and in opening the door between this life and the next. It can be used directly on the skin in a salve and is safe to drink as tea.

✳ **CARAWAY.** Frequently used in baking, caraway has a mild licorice flavor. It promotes a sense of vitality and well-being and aids in clear thinking.

✳ **CHAMOMILE.** This soothing herb is delicious in tea, providing a sense of peace and tranquility. Aids in meditation and gentle rest.

✳ **GARLIC.** For protection—and not just from vampires. Boosts the immune system, as well as your sense of courage.

✳ **LAVENDER.** Helps to find balance and establish communication, including with the greater unknown universe and your own intuition. Aids in meditation and helps you find your own internal wisdom. Safe—and delicious—for consumption.

✳ **LEMON BALM.** Also known as "melissa," this member of the mint family has a distinct lemony scent. It improves mood and mental clarity and can calm anxiety to allow restful sleep. It is delicious and safe to consume.

✳ **MINT.** Certainly delicious and safe to eat, mint energizes, promotes clarity of thought, aids in communication and concentration, and offers good luck!

✳ **MULLEIN.** The clear quartz of herbal healing, mullein is good for respiratory relief, as well as earache, fever, sore throat, and headaches. It is safe to drink.

✳ **MUGWORT.** Helps you connect to the unseen world. Provides wisdom and energy while enhancing psychic abilities.

✳ **ROSE.** Good for the skin due to its anti-inflammatory and antioxidant properties, rose is of course also known for its elegant sense of love.

✳ **ROSEMARY.** This delicious herb aids in concentration, divination, communication, and of course memory. "Rosemary is for remembrance."

✳ **RUE.** Also known as "Herb of Grace," rue is used to promote menstruation, and—paradoxically, maybe—it provides a sense of calm and well-being. Since it does cause menstruation, it can also cause a miscarriage, so do not consume while pregnant and always use in small amounts.

✳ **SAGE.** This herb of wisdom is also good for fertility and can aid in overall health and longevity. It also helps with communication and concentration and is, of course, safe for consumption.

✳ **SAINT JOHN'S WORT.** Encourages strength and willpower while combating depression. It is safe for consumption, but may interact with antidepressants.

✳ **THYME.** This common kitchen herb helps you tap into your inner strength, gives you a sense of renewed energy, and can purify your spirit.

✳ **VALERIAN.** The roots of this pretty plant provide a mild sedative and can also calm anxiety and depression. It is safe to drink as a tea, or you can steep the roots in a neutral alcohol, like vodka, for a stronger dose.

✳ **VERVAIN.** Vervain also helps with anxiety and insomnia and can ease muscle tension while providing a sense of overall well-being. Safe to drink, though it occasionally causes nausea. It does smell very nice.

✳ **WORMWOOD.** This bitter and aromatic plant is one of the foundations for absinthe, so use it sparingly. It is an anti-inflammatory and fever-reducing herb and has been used for divination.

✳ **YARROW.** This lovely and common member of the sunflower family relieves cold and flu symptoms, cramps, and offers a sense of calm and relaxation, while enhancing your psychic abilities.

USING HERBS

Any of the above can be found fresh, dried, or in essential oil form. If you grow your own herbs, you can either use them fresh for tea or making an herbal oil, or you can hang them upside down to dry for two to four weeks.

HERBAL OILS

An herbal oil allows you to preserve your herbs for use long into the winter, and it can be incorporated into a lotion or balm or used as an anointing oil in ritual. And they're exceedingly simple to make: start by chopping your herbs with a knife or bruising them using a mortar and pestle. You want to break past the barrier of the skin to release the oils. Place your herbs in a jar and fill it with the carrier oil of your choice—olive or almond oil work particularly well. Cover the herbs by at least one inch, and leave one inch of space at the top of the container. Close the jar tightly, and allow it to rest for one month, in sunlight if possible. Once the month is up, you can strain the oil through cheesecloth on an as-needed basis, leaving the remaining herbal oil to continue steeping.

ESSENTIAL OILS

Essential oils can serve much the same function as herbal oils, just in a more powerful way. Essential oils are a distillation of the oils of the plant, capturing its aroma as well as its magical properties—literally its "essence." It would take a handful of dried sage to achieve the same power as a drop of sage essential oil, but more importantly, many of the plants mentioned above are kind of hard to find fresh or dried. You can't really get myrrh and frankincense at your local garden center.

However, essential oils can be really expensive. The good news is that there is absolutely no reason to pay top dollar for them. There's no governing body managing the quality of essential oils, and unless you're planning on drinking your essential oils—which you should never, ever do—therapeutic-grade is perfectly safe. Make sure your essential oils are 100 percent undiluted, and be careful using some of them directly on your skin. (Lemon and lime essential oils can cause a sunburn if you spend too long out in the sun).

The aromatherapy practices in this book include creating a blend of essential oils . . . which can be a little intimidating, because how do you know what scents will go well together? No matter the benefits of the individual essential oils, if they don't blend harmoniously, they won't achieve much in the way of aromatherapy. The method for this is much like the theory behind making perfumes: a balanced perfume will contain a top note—with a bright, fresh scent—usually the first thing you smell in a perfume—a middle note—with a warm, occasionally spicy scent—and a base note—with a deeper, earthy scent. These three notes together will create a rich, resonant experience.

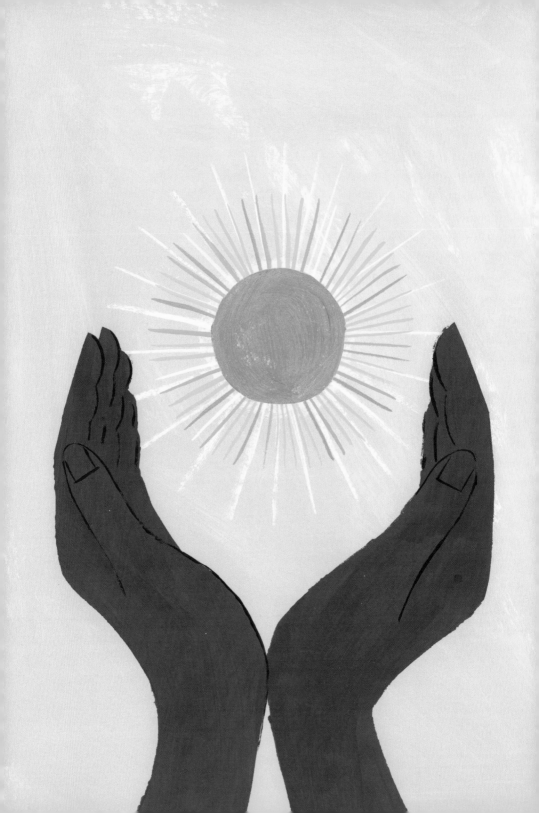

CREATIVITY

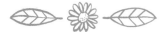

the ability to transcend traditional ideas, rules, patterns, relationships, or the like, and to create meaningful new ideas, forms, methods, or interpretations; originality or imagination

WELL, THAT WAS A BIT OF A MOUTHFUL, as dictionary definitions tend to be. But the kind of creativity we're talking about is complex. It's not just "the ability to create"—a circular definition if ever there was one. It's the ability to look at the established understanding of what is impossible and find a way to make it possible—in essence, magic.

It isn't easy. It requires every piece of our intuition, our resourcefulness, and our inspiration . . . not to mention our courage. Everything in this book has been preparing you for this, helping you to find a space of peace and clarity within—for it is only under those conditions that you can begin to cultivate this kind of creativity.

Let us begin.

Body

Yoga Practice to Tap Into Creative Energy

Creativity comes in many forms. It can be a new perspective, a strength of purpose, playfulness, or a sense of freedom. Each of these poses will help you cultivate an aspect of creativity, bringing them all together into one whole piece.

VIRASANA

(Hero Pose)

If you've been practicing yoga for a while and are comfortable going into the full version of this pose, please do so. Otherwise, come to a kneeling position on your mat. Bring your knees and feet together, and then gently rest back on your heels. Place your palms on your thighs and rotate your shoulders back, raising your chest to the sky. You are the hero of your own story.

MALASANA

(Squat)

Stand at the front of your mat and place your feet at the edges. Turn your toes out so that they spill over onto the floor beneath. Slowly, sink your hips down, pulling your tailbone (your root chakra) toward the earth. Bring your palms into prayer position and press the outside edges of your elbows into your knees, pushing back with your knees into your elbows. Keep your shoulders back and your spine as straight as possible. If your heels come up, that's completely fine. Many women around the world give birth in this position. Stay here for as long as it's comfortable. What will you give birth to?

VIRASANA

MALASANA

GARUDASANA

CAMATKARASANA

SALAMBA
SARVANGASANA

GARUDASANA
(Eagle Pose)

Rise up and stand once more at the front of your mat. Bring your feet together and bend your knees, keeping your feet flat on the mat. Lift your right leg and cross it over your left knee. If you can, hook your right foot around your left ankle. Keep your core tight and find something in front of you to focus on—this will help you balance. If you feel secure, stretch your arms straight out in front of you and cross your right arm beneath the left and work to bring the palms of your hands to touch. Maintain that fierce focus, as well as your control of your lower core and your sacral chakra, the chakra of creativity. Repeat on the other side.

SALAMBA SARVANGASANA
(Shoulder Stand)

Release and come to lie flat on your back. If you want, place a towel or blanket up under your neck to support you in this pose. Bring your knees up to your chest, feeling the stretch in your lower back, the underside of your sacral chakra. Place your hands beneath your hips, and lift your hips up to sky, rolling onto your upper back. When you're ready, straighten your legs, imagining a rope or vine hanging from the sky pulling your feet toward the sun. Support your upper back with your hands, and take a look around you. What does life look like from this new perspective?

CAMATKARASANA
(Wild Thing)

Come into side plank, with the outside edge of your right foot touching the earth and your left foot resting on top. Your right arm is straight, and your left hip arches toward the sky. Your right hand supports your upper body weight. Bring your left foot down behind you, taking some of the weight off of the right foot. Keep the left foot bent and the right foot straight out in front of you. Reach your left arm up and behind you, and arch the chest and hips up to sky. Be wild. Be free. Be open, in every way and to everything.

Sacral Chakra Practice

Svadisthana, the sacral chakra, governs our creativity in all senses of the word. An active, open sacral chakra means that you can access your inspiration and imagination . . . and it is also, by definition, a little sexy. Give yourself permission to turn on that part of yourself. If you feel a little silly or uncomfortable, make sure you're either alone or with someone who can laugh with and explore with you.

Begin by gathering two crystals relating to the sacral chakra, like sunstone, rutilated quartz, carnelian, garnet, ruby, or citrine. They can both be the same, or you can use two different ones—whatever feels right for you. Sit cross-legged on the floor, and place a crystal on each knee, holding them in place with your hands. Keep your spine straight.

Begin to move the chest in a circle, keeping your hips still and your shoulders straight. Bring your rib cage to the right, smooth it across the front and around to the left, and then curve it back. Keep going, around and around. Generate some energy with this motion, stirring up all that has been stuck inside you. Pay attention to the crystals beneath your palms, and feel them heat up.

When you're ready, change direction, smoothing your rib cage to the left, across the front, and pulling your hips and belly button around and to the back. Feel this motion down in your hips, as you keep your tailbone rooted to the floor and your knees down. See if you can make a little dance of this, perhaps bringing in a little rhythm.

Once you've gotten into it a little bit, change direction again and take a deep breath in. On your exhale, chant VAM, "vuuuummmmmmmmmm." Repeat two times more, and then switch direction again, chanting three more times, "vuuuuuummmmmmmmmmm."

Now, begin to slow it down. Move in smaller and smaller circles, feeling as if your body is a ribbon wrapping around a maypole. Eventually, the ribbon will straighten, and your spine will be aligned. Close your eyes, and take three deep, silent breaths.

Divination Tea

This tea serves a dual purpose: to help you divine what could be possible and to give you the energy to make it so. Consume it first thing in the morning, ideally while sitting in the warmth of the sun.

Mix a total of half a teaspoon of the following herbs for divination:

Yarrow   **Wormwood**   **Sage**   **Mugwort**   **Lavender**

Add to your mixture a total of a half a teaspoon of the following herbs for energy:

Thyme   **Mint**   **Caraway**

Pour some just-boiled water over your herb mixture, and allow it to steep for three to five minutes. As you sip your tea, jot down any ideas that come to you, however far-fetched or "impossible." Some of them will be absurd, some of them will be boring, some of them will be practical, and some of them will be inspired. All of them will tell you something you need to know.

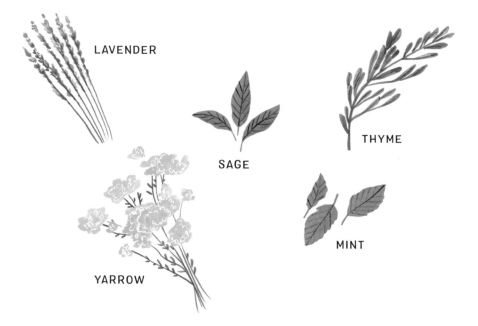

LAVENDER

SAGE

THYME

MINT

YARROW

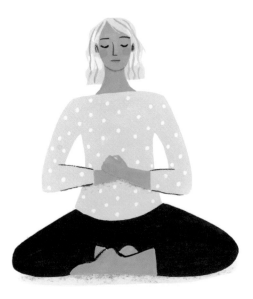

Solar Plexus Chakra Practice

Manipura is your chakra of power. Your solar plexus rests right beneath the rib cage, at your upper core. Take a moment and find that space, that arch at the top center, beneath your ribs. Tighten it and massage it. It feels like a literal circle, like a firm disc of energy. You need this energy, this power, to *do something* with all the creativity you've made space for.

Gather a crystal that interacts well with your solar plexus chakra, like tigereye, pyrite, yellow jasper, or mookaite. Sit comfortably, but in a way that engages your core slightly and keeps your spine straight—a cross-legged seat will work, or you might consider hero pose, as described on page 106. Hold your crystal in your left hand and close your fist around it. Bring your left fist to rest right on your solar plexus chakra, and cover your fist with your right hand.

This pranayama, or breath practice, is called Kapalabhati, also known as skull shining breath or breath of fire. It can take a bit of getting used to, as it asks you to breathe in a very different way. Ordinarily, we put some energy into the inhale, but the exhale just kind of happens on its own, passively. It's not like we have to push the air out. In Kapalabhati, that is reversed: we forcefully push the air out, and the inhale remains passive.

Keeping your fists in place, take a deep inhale through your nose. Push the air out in small bursts, also through your nose, using the muscles beneath your fists to exhale. You'll make a sound like a piston, pumping up and down. Find a rhythm that works for you, and allow the inhale to come when you need it. If you lose your rhythm, just come back to it.

Eventually, your core will start to burn, and you'll want to stop. When that happens, continue for just a little bit longer. When you stop, open your hands, and take a deep inhale. On your exhale, chant RAM, "ruuuuuum-mmmmmmmmmm."

Mermaid Bath

Think about lying in a bath with a glass of wine, reading a book or resting with cucumbers on your eyes. Could anything be more relaxing? And often that's enough, but for a more powerful ritual, add in some intention and some ancestral connection with magic and the divine.

Cultures all across the world and throughout history have created bathing rituals intended to help find peace. The Greeks, Romans, Turks, Finns, Japanese, Balinese, Mayans—there are so many, and their rituals are often in honor of or inspired by the deities or spirits of their culture. For instance, the Yoruban goddess Yemayá is an orisha, or a human spirit incarnation from Santería traditions. She is a goddess of water and of women and is often depicted as a mermaid. Her mythology says that when her water broke when giving birth, it caused a great flood creating rivers and streams. The first humans were born from her womb. She governs deep secrets, ancient wisdom, and feminine creativity. This ritual is inspired by her, but it is also an invitation to explore the rituals created by your own ancestors, by the gods and goddesses in whose domain you live.

You'll need:

- o Blue or white flower petals
- o Fresh mint or mint essential oil
- o 20–30 drops of a blend of ylang-ylang and ginger essential oils
- o 1–2 cups sea salt
- o A large seashell
- o Almond, jojoba, or coconut oil
- o Blue or white candles

Cleanse yourself with cool water, wiping down your face and arms and feet. Fill a bath with hot water, but not so hot that you can't immediately immerse yourself into it. Add the first four ingredients to your bath and fill the seashell with your chosen oil. Light your candles, whispering a prayer or intention as you do so. Stir the water counterclockwise to dissolve the salts, creating a whirlpool of the herbs and flowers. Step into the bath and close your eyes. Immerse your hair, your body, even your face if you like.

When you emerge, dip a finger into the oil resting in the seashell. Anoint your temples, your eyelids, your sacral chakra, your crown chakra, and your wrists and feet. Smooth the oil down your legs, and watch it float up, separate from and yet contained by the water.

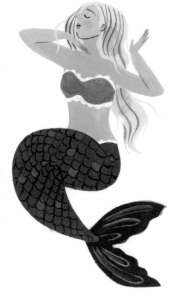

Stay in the bath for as long as you like, allowing yourself to soak up feminine creativity. Feel the warmth of the water. Feel the buoyancy of the salt. Notice the way the flower petals and herbs brush up against your skin as the water moves with you. *Be sensual.*

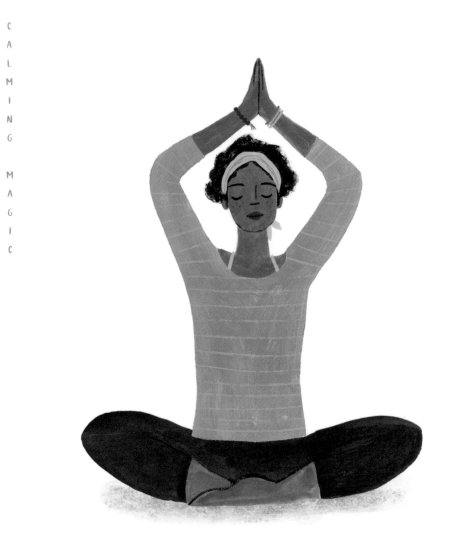

Crown Chakra Practice

Sahasrara is a special chakra. Some descriptions say it actually resides just *above* the top of your head, floating there. We do, of course, have energy fields around us. You know that feeling when someone is standing just a little too close to you and you want to reach back to the nineties and say "get off my bubble?" That bubble is the boundary of your energy field, and sahasrara exists at the top edge.

It makes a certain amount of sense that your crown chakra would float magically in the ether, as your crown chakra represents your connection with magic, possibility, and the divine.

Take a moment to find a crystal whose vibrations resonate with sahasrara, like sugilite, opal, amethyst, kyanite, clear quartz, celestite, or apophyllite. Hold it between your palms and rub it between them, as if you're rolling a ball of dough to make cookies. Generate some heat and energy, and once you feel the crystal grow warm, set it aside.

Stand with your feet together, or find a comfortable seat, keeping your shoulders back. Keep your chin level, as you don't want your gaze reaching up toward the heavens. Instead, imagine your crown chakra hovering there. Inhale and spread your arms, reaching them up toward the sky. Clap them together—this is called *Jai*, meaning "victory." Use it as a celebration of sahasrara, of your connection with magic. Keep your palms together in prayer, and lower them to rest above your heart.

Inhale and reach your arms out and up. *Jai!* Bring them back down in a prayer pose over your heart. Namaste.

Flow in this way again and again. Follow your own instincts. You can do it three times, five times, even twenty times. Ask yourself what is being asked of you. Sahasrara will tell you.

When you feel complete, keep your hands in prayer. Take a deep breath in, and as you exhale, chant OHM, "ooohhhhhhhhhhhmmmmmmmm."

Release your hands. You may feel a little flush of energy, of joy. If you do, lean into it. If you can, try a headstand or handstand, or even a cartwheel. If that isn't your jam, put on a song that you can never, ever help but sing along to. Hug someone you love.

Mind

Altar Practice

Wipe the slate of your altar clean. Instead of simply tidying and judiciously considering and putting aside anything that no longer feels quite right, take everything off and start from scratch. Just as rearranging your living room can make your house feel like an entirely new home, reenvisioning your altar can be a shot of creative adrenaline.

Begin by selecting a new centerpiece. You may consider an image or other representation of a goddess of creativity:

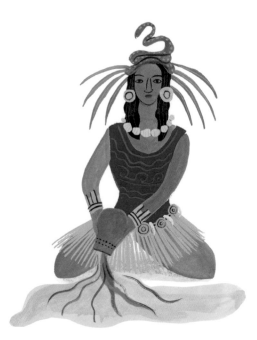

- Danu, the mother of the Irish gods and of the Tuatha Dé Danann, who are sometimes called the fey, is a goddess of fertility and also of art, skill, knowledge, and wisdom. It is said that the mists of Ireland are her loving embrace.

- Ixchel is a Mayan goddess; she was given her name in the sixteenth century, but she may date to as early as 2000 BCE. She is the goddess of fertility, love, the moon, and medicine. She is often shown pouring out a jar of water.

- Saraswati is the Hindu goddess of art, music, knowledge, and learning. In one legend, she is said to have saved the world from an all-consuming fire called Vadavagni by transforming into a river.

You'll note that each of these deities, along with many other gods and goddesses associated with creativity, has something to do with water. To enhance the inspiration given by water, you may consider placing an open bowl of water on your altar or a jar of rain or river water.

Now, fire and water typically do not get along (Saraswati certainly knew that). However, both are symbols of creative energy, and your altar is capable of holding more than one idea—as are you. Balance your water with some incense, like dragon's blood, amber, peppermint, or cardamom.

Aromatherapy Practice

For a blend that sparks your intuition and invites energy and inspiration, choose from the following:

TOP NOTES

- BERGAMOT. Used in Ayurvedic and Italian folk medicine traditions, this light citrusy scent is popular in the perfume industry. It is known to aid in motivation and inspiration.

- EUCALYPTUS. Historically used for respiratory ailments, eucalyptus also provides energy, focus, and optimism.

✳ PIÑON. The clear, spicy scent of pine can help you envision and create a plan for moving forward.

✳ JUNIPER. This spicier, more resinous piney aroma supports your overall energy and focus.

✳ LEMON. If you need to see with fresh eyes, lemon can do that for you.

MIDDLE NOTES

✳ CARDAMOM. This spicy, warm-sweet scent provides you with uplifting comfort. Be careful applying it directly to your skin, as it can cause irritation.

✳ KUNZEA. From a pink and white flowering tree from Australia and Tasmania, kunzea essential oil is somehow both woodsy and herbal. Its cleansing properties help you to feel both relaxed and inspired.

✳ THYME. Thyme can give you both energy and a sense of purpose.

✳ NEROLI. Sharply floral, neroli can help you feel more centered and open to inspiration.

BASE NOTES

✳ CEDARWOOD. Sweetly woodsy, cedarwood provides comfort and a gentle boost.

✳ SPIKENARD. This heavy, earthy fragrance finds its way into perfumes as often as patchouli does. Its grounding qualities help you to feel centered.

✳ CLOVE. Invigorating, energizing, and cleansing, clove essential oil's spicy, autumnal scent will add an earthy quality to your blend.

Combine one part base note, two parts middle note, and one part top note. Add the mixture to an essential oil diffuser, or you can create a perfume oil by mixing it with an unscented carrier like sweet almond or grapeseed oil.

Meditation Practice

Meditation practice can often feel intimidating, and it's hard to know if we're doing it "right." Of course, there is no right or wrong way to do it, but it does feel that way sometimes. The stages of meditation described on page 65—dharana, dhyana, and samadhi—can feel unreachable, unless you're a guru or something.

This simply isn't true. Again, samadhi, or enlightenment, is a goal, rather than something most people experience—although it is something anyone can find at any time, even if fleetingly. But if you've practiced the meditations for peace and clarity, you have already reached the stage of dharana. In this meditation, we will explore dhyana. It will take a bit longer than usual, so make sure you have plenty of undisturbed time.

Start by putting on some meditative music—there are all sorts of options available online or on various music apps. This may not be traditional, but it certainly isn't "cheating"—music has a profound impact on the brain and can help you get out of your usual thought patterns. Light some incense—you may consider amber, benzoin, myrrh, palo santo, wormwood, or frankincense.

Then, begin as always by finding a comfortable seat. Sit cross-legged, and observe the way your legs naturally rest. Is the right ankle on top of the left? If so, switch it. Test yourself a little by sitting in a way that feels a little awkward. By pushing yourself outside of what you're used to, you can find your way past the limits you have set for yourself.

Start with some pranayama. Inhale for a count of four, hold for a count of four, exhale for a count of four, and rest for a count of four. Repeat this process until you have found your rhythm, and then stop counting and simply breathe in this way. If you find yourself returning to worries of the day and other clamoring thoughts, just return to your count for a while. Give yourself as much time as you need.

Once you've settled into this rhythm, allow your mind to drift. You may find your imagination sparking with images, sounds, even sensations. Receive whatever comes to you, without seeking.

When you're ready to come out of your trance state, do it slowly. Gently move your fingers and toes, and roll your neck carefully before opening your eyes.

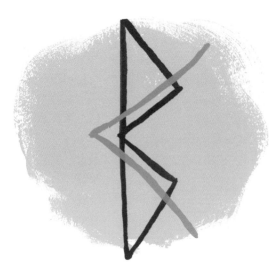

Rune Spell

Create a talisman—something you can keep where you will always see it or carry with you. You can simply draw or paint a rune and paste it above your dresser or at your desk. You can write it on a piece of paper and fold it up small to fit in a locket. You could carve it into a piece of wood to keep in your pocket. Create something with it that feels right for you.

Consider a combination of the following runes:

* Kenaz, for inspiration and creativity

* Wunjo, for the joy we find in work that moves us

* Berkano, for creative energy

* Laguz, for mystery and imagination

* Inguz, for the seed of an idea

You can blend them together in any way you choose—the symbol pictured is just one interpretation. It is entirely up to you, and you will power your talisman with the creativity you bring to it.

Feng Shui Support

If you haven't explored the baguas, this is a good time to start. What sort of creativity do you want to invite? We need creativity in all areas of our lives, whether it's at work, in our relationships, with our families, or with what we want to offer the world. Where do you most need creativity at this moment?

Once you've settled on a location, add the element of wood. Ordinarily this can take many forms, as much of the furniture we all use is made of wood, but in this case you want to focus on *living* wood, something green and growing. If your thumb is incurably black, try something hardy like succulents, pathos plants, or philodendrons. This will invite life and literal creation into your space.

Complement that with some water; a little mystery will bring forth your intuition. A mirror set where it will reflect the light from a window can help expand your mind.

While fire and water don't exactly get along, fire's energy is necessary to spark wood's creativity. Consider how a forest fire can promote growth, but remember that this fire must be controlled. A small candle or a red throw pillow will suffice.

Creativity Tincture

A tincture is a potent blend of herbs steeped in alcohol. You use them more often than you think. Vanilla extract? That's a tincture, and it's quite easy to make yourself. For this particular tincture, gather the following herbs:

Caraway, for clear thinking

Lavender, for internal wisdom

Mugwort, to help you connect with the unseen

Sage, for wisdom

Thyme, for energy

Wormwood, for divination

Yarrow, to enhance psychic abilities

You will need a tablespoon of each. If any are dried, crush them a little between your palms or in a mortar and pestle. If any are fresh, chop them lightly, bruising them a little to release their juices. Mix all your herbs together and place them in a jar. Cover your herbs with alcohol—either Everclear or vodka will work, and there's no need to use the good stuff. Allow your mixture to steep for one month in a dark place.

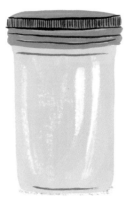

When the month has passed, strain your tincture through a cheesecloth or paper towel into a dark glass container. It will keep for a year or more. When you're in need of a creative boost, consume a teaspoon's worth.

Heart

Crystal Grid for Creativity

Start by finding your way outside and collecting wildflowers. Dandelions, Queen Anne's lace, daisies, buttercups, cherry blossoms, cornflowers, violets, yarrow, milkweed, even thistles—whatever is growing, use that. If it's autumn, collect leaves or acorns, and if it's winter, pluck some evergreen or ivy. You can always find *something*, even in a city, if you look.

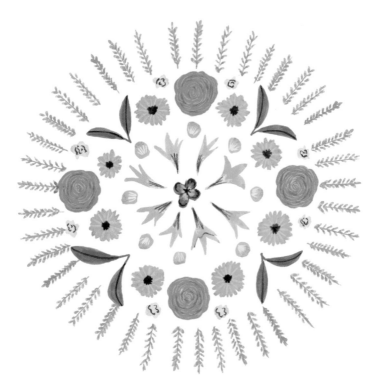

Then gather a selection of the following crystals. There's no need to find an exact number—you can work with whatever you have on hand.

Agate	Bronzite	Jade	Ruby
Amazonite	Calcite	Lapis lazuli	Rutilated quartz
Amethyst	Carnelian	Mookaite	Sardonyx
Aventurine	Chrysocolla	Opal	Sunstone
Bloodstone	Garnet	Peridot	

Spread out your flowers and crystals, sorting them by color, type, size—whatever you want. For this mandala, there is no exact plan, no layout. Have fun with this, interspersing your crystals with your flowers in whatever way appeals to you.

Tarot Reading to Find Your Purpose

This is an unusual tarot reading, in that it isn't for a single moment, but for always—or at least, for as long as you need this reading to be true. It is easiest to do this reading once you've spent a fair amount of time with your cards and gotten to know them a little bit. Your cards will take on your energy, and you will begin to understand each other on a deeper level.

Lay out each card faceup. They don't need to be in any sort of order, but you should be able to see all of them.

Begin by taking away the cards that do not speak to you. Hardly anyone wants to identify with Death, or the Tower, or the Eight of Cups. Set aside any card that isn't what you want.

Examine what's left. Now it's time to consider what draws you, what feels like who you truly are. Are you the Empress? Are you the Queen of Wands? Are you the Star? Take your time and consider each card. You may

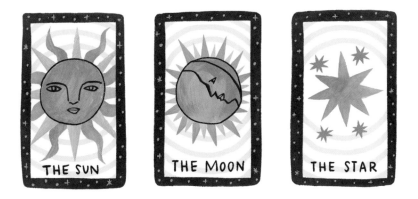

THE SUN   THE MOON   THE STAR

have trouble settling on just one, as we are all complicated people and may not align exactly with one single archetype. In that case, consider what you *want* to be right now. What aspect of yourself do you most want to explore?

When you've found your card, place it on your altar for a while. Let its energy permeate your altar, and infuse the card with the energy of your altar. The next time you go to do a reading—really, every reading you do from now on—this card will have a deeper meaning. It will represent *you*, as you truly are.

Lunar Ritual

Scrying is a form of divination done by gazing—most often into a bowl of water. It is mentioned in the Book of Genesis, as well as in many, many folkloric traditions. It can be performed at any time, but for our purposes it should be done on the night of the full moon.

Select a large bowl, like a salad or serving bowl. Earthenware, ceramic, or wood is best. Fill your bowl with water and carry it to a place where you can see the moonlight reflected in the water. If you can arrange your bowl so that it captures the moon's face in the water, all the better, but this isn't strictly necessary.

Add twenty-eight drops of some combination of the following essential oils:

Calendula   Mugwort   Rosemary   Wormwood   Yarrow

Turn out all your lights, so that the water reflects only the moon. Lean over your bowl and inhale deeply, breathing in the fragrance of your essential oils. Let your body and mind come to rest. Observe the motion of the water as it moves with your breath, with any rumblings from a car driving by, with the heartbeat of the earth. Eventually, allow your eyes to soften and blur, but keep them focused on the water.

As you enter a trance state as described on page 119, you will begin to notice something in the water. It may be just a word, or an image, or even an entire scene. Let it come.

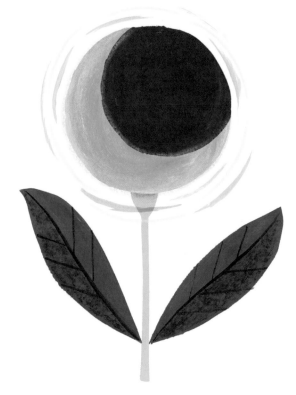

When you have finished, dip a jar into the water and save it, putting it away in a safe place until the next full moon. Before you go to sleep, write in your journal about what it was that you saw, and for each night until the next full moon, continue to journal, inquiring further about your vision. On the night of the following full moon, retrieve your jar and anoint your eyelids with its water, keeping the knowledge you received close.

Candle Spell

To live as ourselves in the world openly and without fear of judgment, complete in our own power, takes courage. Whenever fear begins to bite at your heels, turn to this spell.

Select a red candle. Take small knife and etch the following runes (see page 14) into its sides:

Uruz   Sowilo   Dagaz

Crush a clove of garlic and rub its oils on the candle. If it's available, sprinkle some Saint John's wort on as well, taking care to avoid the wick. Surround the base of your candle with the following crystals:

Agate   Bloodstone   Sardonyx   Tigereye

When you're ready, light your candle. Watch it flicker, and raise a palm to rest above the flame, so that its heat forms a sharp point pressing into your palm. Bring your palm to your heart, and feel the heat there.

You have the support of the earth, of those who have come before you, of nature, and of the elements. You have everything you need. You *are* everything you need.

Let your fire burn.

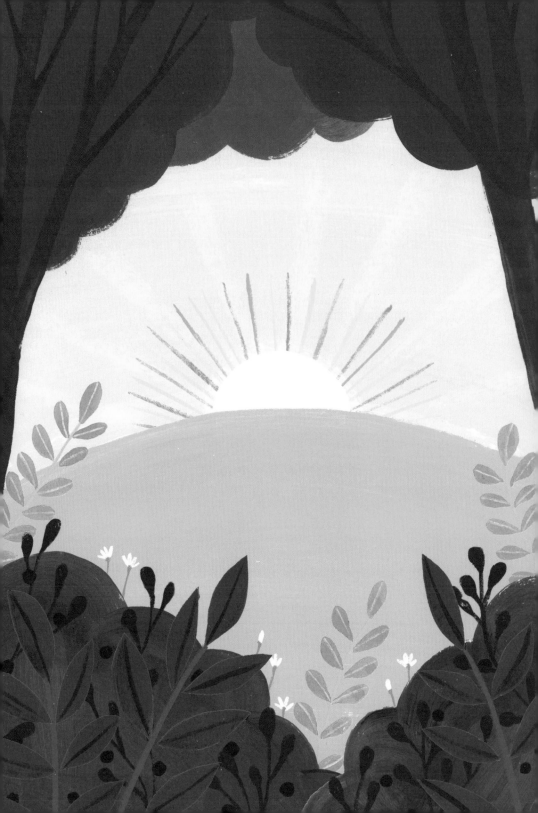

CONCLUSION

We have ended this book in a very different place from where we began. The promise of peace offered in *Calming Magic* is not one to be taken lightly, for peace is something we continually seek and refine.

But it is not a state of being that we can ever maintain for long. Inevitably, some internal or external force disturbs that peace. And this is just as it should be—if we were to live a life undisturbed, it would not be much of a life at all. Consider, for a moment, what it would be like to always be calm, to never feel the vibrancy of joy, the tightness of anger, or even the heaviness of disappointment that is an occasional result of the pull of desire. These are emotions that we must not only experience, but celebrate. They are part of the experience of life, and they are magical.

Whenever you need it, you can come back to that place of calm and find that sense of clarity. It is essential to be able to remove yourself from your stressors and take a break—but don't stay there. Be a disturbance in the world from time to time. Spark those around you out of their own calm if it has stagnated. The image that comes to mind when we think of calm is often of a ripple in a pond. But remember, that ripple was created by something that splashed into the water.

ACKNOWLEDGMENTS

Thank you to Maile for letting me borrow her crystals and tinctures, and to Dave for letting me spread runes and tarot cards everywhere, and for keeping the fire going when I forget. Thank you to Heather for talking balms with me, to Yamile for Yémaya, and to Tulani for being a soul sister. Thank you to Mom and Dad for solstices and poetry.

Shannon Fabricant, I really love this one! It was a joy to write, and thank you so much. I'm so happy to walk this road with you. Susan Van Horn, you are a master of design, and I am grateful for you every day. Penelope Dullaghan, your stunning illustrations have made this book a work of art—thank you so much. Thank you to the hawk-eyed Ashley Benning, and to Kristin Kiser, Amy Cianfrone, and the entire Running Press team. You are all magical, and I'm so grateful for all that you do.

INDEX

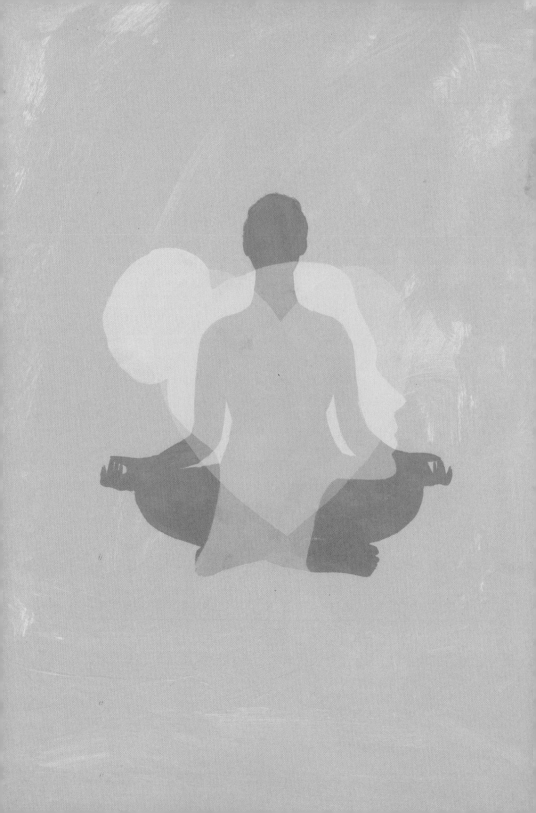